Dr Shahid Aziz (MBChB, _____ ___ __ North Bristol NHS Trust and the B. _____ in a large teaching hospital looking after patie _____ conditions, including hypertension, heart attacks _____ His particular interest is the treatment of coronary artery _____ with coronary angioplasty and stents. His research interests include _____ mization of angioplasty results, and he has published several papers in the field of interventional cardiology. He plays a leading role in medical teaching through Bristol University, and on the General Medical Council as a member of the review panel for cardiology specialist registration. His website is at <www.bristolcardiologist.com>.

Dr Zara Aziz is a GP working in a large and busy urban practice in Bristol. She has interests in cardiovascular health, family medicine and disease prevention. She is involved in medical education and trains junior doctors to become GPs. She is a keen medical writer and writes for a number of publications, including a 'Doctor's orders' column for The Guardian.

Overcoming Common Problems Series

Selected titles

A full list of titles is available from Sheldon Press,
36 Causton Street, London SW1P 4ST and on our website at
www.sheldonpress.co.uk

Breast Cancer: Your treatment choices
Dr Terry Priestman

Chronic Fatigue Syndrome: What you need to know about CFS/ME
Dr Megan A. Arroll

Cider Vinegar
Margaret Hills

Coping Successfully with Chronic Illness: Your healing plan
Neville Shone

Coping Successfully with Hiatus Hernia
Dr Tom Smith

Coping with Difficult Families
Dr Jane McGregor and Tim McGregor

Coping with Epilepsy
Dr Pamela Crawford and Fiona Marshall

Coping with Guilt
Dr Windy Dryden

Coping with Liver Disease
Mark Greener

Coping with Memory Problems
Dr Sallie Baxendale

Coping with Obsessive Compulsive Disorder
Professor Kevin Gournay, Rachel Piper and Professor Paul Rogers

Coping with the Psychological Effects of Illness
Dr Fran Smith, Dr Carina Eriksen and Professor Robert Bor

Coping with Schizophrenia
Professor Kevin Gournay and Debbie Robson

Coping with Thyroid Disease
Mark Greener

Depressive Illness: The curse of the strong
Dr Tim Cantopher

The Empathy Trap: Understanding antisocial personalities
Dr Jane McGregor and Tim McGregor

Epilepsy: Complementary and alternative treatments
Dr Sallie Baxendale

The Fibromyalgia Healing Diet
Christine Craggs-Hinton

Fibromyalgia: Your treatment guide
Christine Craggs-Hinton

Hay Fever: How to beat it
Dr Paul Carson

Helping Elderly Relatives
Jill Eckersley

The Holistic Health Handbook
Mark Greener

How to Eat Well When You Have Cancer
Jane Freeman

How to Stop Worrying
Dr Frank Tallis

Invisible Illness: Coping with misunderstood conditions
Dr Megan A. Arroll and Professor Christine P. Dancey

Living with Complicated Grief
Professor Craig A. White

Living with Fibromyalgia
Christine Craggs-Hinton

Living with Hearing Loss
Dr Don McFerran, Lucy Handscomb and Dr Cherilee Rutherford

Living with IBS
Nuno Ferreira and David T. Gillanders

Overcoming Fear: With mindfulness
Deborah Ward

Overcoming Stress
Professor Robert Bor, Dr Carina Eriksen and Dr Sara Chaudry

Overcoming Worry and Anxiety
Dr Jerry Kennard

Physical Intelligence: How to take charge of your weight
Dr Tom Smith

The Self-Esteem Journal
Alison Waines

The Stroke Survival Guide
Mark Greener

Ten Steps to Positive Living
Dr Windy Dryden

Treating Arthritis: The drug-free way
Margaret Hills and Christine Horner

Treating Arthritis: The supplements guide
Julia Davies

Understanding Yourself and Others: Practical ideas from the world of coaching
Bob Thomson

When Someone You Love Has Depression: A handbook for family and friends
Barbara Baker

Overcoming Common Problems

Understanding High Blood Pressure

DR SHAHID AZIZ
and
DR ZARA AZIZ

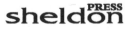

First published in Great Britain in 2015

Sheldon Press
36 Causton Street
London SW1P 4ST
www.sheldonpress.co.uk

British Library Cataloguing-in-Publication Data
A catalogue record for this book is available from the British Library

ISBN 978-1-84709-326-4
eBook ISBN 978-1-84709-327-1

Typeset by Fakenham Prepress Solutions, Fakenham, Norfolk NR21 8NN
First printed in Great Britain by Ashford Colour Press
Subsequently digitally reprinted in Great Britain

eBook by Fakenham Prepress Solutions, Fakenham, Norfolk NR21 8NN

Produced on paper from sustainable forests

*This book is dedicated to our family
for their boundless love and support*

Contents

Note to the reader

This is not a medical book and is not intended to replace advice from your doctor. Consult your pharmacist or doctor if you believe you have any of the symptoms described, and if you think you might need medical help.

Introduction

I am a consultant cardiologist working in a busy city hospital. In my clinical work, I see many patients who have high blood pressure. Patients with high blood pressure can end up in hospital in two different ways. First, they may be admitted when they are acutely unwell with a heart attack, heart failure or stroke. This can be due to undiagnosed high blood pressure (hypertension) or because they have hypertension that needs to be controlled better. These patients can be extremely ill, especially if they have had a severe stroke, which is the most disabling complication of high blood pressure.

Second, patients with complex hypertension are referred to my clinic by their GPs. The GPs may have found it difficult to select the correct drug combination to control these patients' blood pressure or the patients could be intolerant to medications. Sometimes young patients also need specialist investigations, just in case there is an underlying condition that is causing their high blood pressure.

Not everyone with high blood pressure ends up in hospital. For every person I see, there are many more people who have high blood pressure that goes undetected for months or even years. As high blood pressure seldom causes symptoms, an estimated 35 per cent of people with high blood pressure are unaware that they have it. This is why it's important to get your blood pressure checked regularly – and it is even more important if you belong to a group of people who are at high risk of having high blood pressure; for example, those people who have a parent or other close relative with high blood pressure, or people who are heavy smokers, overweight or take no exercise.

Of course, hypertension is not restricted to those people and can affect anybody, which is all the more reason to make sure that your blood pressure is routinely monitored. If you discover that you do have high blood pressure, it is vital that your GP takes action to treat it to prevent the distressing complications it can cause. High blood pressure is one of the most preventable conditions, but it is also very treatable, with effective drug and lifestyle therapies that can prevent complications. However, to successfully manage high blood pressure, you need to take responsibility for it and be involved in your own treatment. This is not always understood or accepted, as those people diagnosed with high blood pressure may not feel that they are not ill as such, and may be reluctant to accept medical treatment. High blood pressure is a 'silent' condition and may not cause any symptoms for many years, so people need support and guidance from healthcare professionals to explain why it needs to be treated. Untreated high blood pressure can result in severe organ damage, including kidney failure, stroke or heart disease. Many people may not want to take medications that can have potential side effects, when they actually feel well. This means that some people do not take their medications regularly and find it difficult to persist with the healthy lifestyle changes recommended by their GPs. Persuading people to comply with treatment is a major challenge in the management of hypertension.

The aim of this book is to summarise, for the public, the current medical knowledge on the diagnosis and treatment of high blood pressure. I will discuss what high blood pressure means, how it is detected, what the risks associated with hypertension are, and best treatment options. Hopefully, by increasing public awareness of the problems and treatment of high blood pressure, we can reduce the substantial health problems that this condition causes.

1

Hypertension: the facts

Hypertension is very common especially as you get older

Hypertension (high blood pressure) is a major public health problem that affects more than one billion people worldwide.

- In the UK, 31.5 per cent of all men and 29 per cent of all women have high blood pressure.
- One in three adults with hypertension is not receiving treatment, as hypertension is not always diagnosed.
- One in two people with hypertension do not have adequate blood pressure control.
- The proportion of the population who have hypertension rises with increasing age; while only 10–20 per cent of people aged 35–44 years have hypertension, 60–70 per cent of people aged 65–74 years have it.
- Men and women who live until they are 85 have a 90 per cent chance of developing hypertension, so most people will develop high blood pressure if they live long enough.
- In the USA, 78 million people, which is approximately one in three adults, have been diagnosed with high blood pressure and the estimated annual cost to treat them is 90 billion dollars.

Over their lifetimes, hypertension affects men and women in equal numbers, although it is more common in women as they get older than men (Table 1).

The number of people with hypertension is predicted to increase by more than 50 per cent over the next 20 years. This is because of the increase in the number of people leading lifestyles that are unhealthy because they involve being less physically active, eating high-calorie and high-salt diets, drinking more alcohol, and becoming obese. The good news is that these lifestyle changes are what we call modifiable risk factors, and it is possible for people to implement a healthier lifestyle (Chapters 9 and 10

Table 1 Hypertension in men and women in different age groups

Age	Men (%)	Women (%)
20–34	11.1	6.8
35–44	25.1	19.0
45–54	37.1	35.2
55–64	54.0	53.3
65–74	64.0	69.3
75 and older	66.7	78.5
All	34.1	32.7

Source Heart disease and stroke statistics – 2013 update: a report from the American Heart Association. *Circulation* 2013; **127**:e6–245.[1]

give advice on how to do it). GPs and practice nurses can also offer advice.

Hypertension is the leading risk factor for many diseases

High blood pressure is the number one global risk factor for premature disease and carries a higher risk for this than smoking and alcohol consumption. High blood pressure has a substantial impact on the quality of many lives and is involved in heart disease, stroke, kidney failure and dementia. Around half of all people with heart disease and three-quarters of all those who have had a stroke have high blood pressure. Hypertension is the second most common cause for kidney failure that requires dialysis; diabetes is the most common cause for this. Most people diagnosed with high blood pressure are often obese, have high blood cholesterol levels and frequently develop diabetes, which are all risk factors for heart disease. This combination of risk factors, which is often referred to as metabolic syndrome, greatly increases the chances of heart disease and stroke.

How do you know if your blood pressure is high?

High blood pressure is often referred to as 'the silent epidemic' because it does not cause any symptoms until organ damage is apparent. GP surgeries and home monitoring programmes need to provide routine blood pressure readings for diagnosis and GP surgeries need to provide effective treatments for high blood pressure. In the UK, blood pressure checks are now a routine part of NHS health checks and everyone aged between 40 to 74, who do not have heart disease or previous stroke, should get a health check every five years. This involves completing a medical history, having a blood pressure check and routine blood tests so that GPs can calculate each person's risk of heart disease.

The doctors and nurses in GP surgeries lead the way with screening and treatments for hypertension and only a small proportion of patients with high blood pressure are referred to hospital specialists, such as myself, for further investigation and treatment. If you are aged over 40 and have not had a health check recently that included measuring your blood pressure, then you should see your GP to request one. Many pharmacists also now provide a service to check blood pressure. Pharmacists can also advise on purchasing automated blood pressure monitors that are accurate and relatively inexpensive and can be used at home.

We need to look after people with high blood pressure better

Despite the availability of medications that effectively lower blood pressure and the relative ease of monitoring blood pressure, a significant proportion of people with high blood pressure are not identified in the first place. This is because large numbers of the population do not regularly see health professionals. Also, up to half of all people who are being treated for high blood pressure do not reach their target blood pressure levels (see Chapter 8), as people need to have the motivation to take the prescribed medication and make changes to their lifestyles. It is understandable that many of us do not like taking tablets when it does not make us feel better. High blood pressure is different to other conditions, such as arthritis or angina where effective treatment improves quality of life, because if your blood pressure is high, often there are no obvious signs or symptoms at all. There are no unpleasant symptoms to be alleviated by drugs, although you may sometimes experience symptoms, such as a headache, with high blood pressure. This means that drugs for hypertension are often prescribed to prevent other diseases, which doesn't meet the perception of medicine as a cure for an existing, troublesome condition.

What is blood pressure?

Before we can look at how best to manage blood pressure, it is important to understand the term 'blood pressure'. The *Oxford Dictionary* defines pressure as a *'physical force'*. A useful working definition for blood pressure is: the force in the circulation that pushes blood around the body.

All the cells in our bodies need a continuous supply of arterial blood, which carries oxygen and nutrients. A constant forward pressure is needed in the circulation to keep the blood flowing, and ensure that the organs and tissues remain healthy. Blood pressure is that forward pressure in our circulation. The pumping action of the heart generates this pressure that drives oxygen-rich blood to every cell in the body.

Cardiac output as a measure of heart function

The heart is an amazing muscular pump that generates the force required to push blood around your circulation. Each day the heart beats about 100,000 times at an average rate of 70 beats per minute. This equates to around 38 million beats per year and over 2.5 billion times for a lifetime of 70 years. It is incredible to think

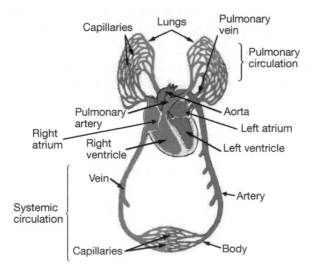

Figure 1 The circulatory system

that your heart can achieve this level of work without needing repair of any sort.

The right-hand side of the heart pumps blood to the lungs where carbon dioxide is removed and oxygen is restored to the blood. The oxygenated blood is then returned to the muscular left ventricle of the heart, which then pumps the blood to the body's vital organs and tissues. With each heartbeat, blood travels down small blood vessels called capillaries that supply the tissues. If lined up side-by-side, the estimated length of the circulatory system would be more than 50,000 miles (Figure 1).

Stroke volume

The force of the contraction of the heart can be measured as the stroke volume: this is the volume of blood that the heart ejects with every contraction that it makes. The average stroke volume is around 70 millilitres and if this figure is multiplied by the heart rate, it gives the cardiac output, which is approximately 5 litres per minute. Blood pressure is a combination of the force and rate of the heartbeat and the vascular resistance, that is, the resistance of the blood vessels to this force. This means that any increases in heart rate, stroke volume or vascular resistance will push blood pressure higher. In practice, the most common cause of high blood pressure is increased vascular resistance.

Blood pressure = force and rate of heartbeat × vascular resistance

What is vascular resistance?

The circulation of blood in the arteries involves a series of tubes of decreasing diameters carrying blood from the heart to the tissues. Artery walls have elastic and muscular tissue that allows them to stretch and absorb some of the force of the pumping blood with each heartbeat. The circular layer of muscle around the arteries can also change the width (diameter) of the arteries. The combined length of tubing in the arterial circulation produces a vascular resistance that has to be overcome for the blood to reach the cells.

Arterioles are the small arteries at the end of the circulation that branch out to supply the tiny blood vessels (capillaries) in the tissues. The arterioles have a relatively thick muscular wall and are

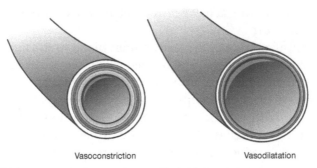

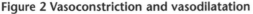

Vasoconstriction   Vasodilatation

Figure 2 Vasoconstriction and vasodilatation

some of the most highly regulated blood vessels in the circulation. They contribute most to the total vascular resistance and are constantly changing size to speed up or slow down tissue blood flow. The diameter of these resistance arterioles is under continuous regulation via a complex system of chemical and electrical nerve impulses (Figure 2).

- Vasoconstriction (a decrease in blood vessel diameter) occurs when the muscular layer in the arterial wall contracts. This increases vascular resistance.
- Vasodilatation (an increase in blood vessel diameter) occurs when the muscular layer in the arterial wall relaxes. This decreases vascular resistance.

Adrenaline is a powerful hormone that reduces the diameter of arteries (constriction), increases heart rate, and strengthens heart contractions; all of which leads to an increase in blood pressure. This is why adrenaline is used in medical emergencies where the blood pressure is dangerously low, such as after a cardiac arrest (when the heart stops) or anaphylaxis (a severe and life-threatening allergic reaction).

Most causes of high blood pressure are linked to an increase in the vascular resistance due to a decrease in the diameter of blood vessels (vasoconstriction) and many of the drug treatments for hypertension lower blood pressure by causing dilatation of blood vessels and, therefore, a decrease in the vascular resistance (Figure 3).

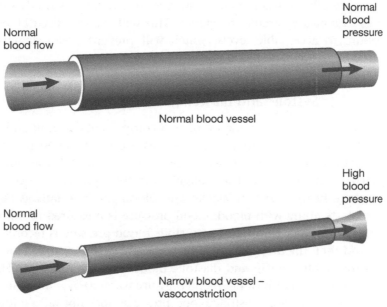

Figure 3 Diagram showing high blood pressure due to
vasoconstriction and high vascular resistance

Can low blood pressure be a problem?

A very low blood pressure can also cause problems. Sometimes
heart function abnormalities will cause a very slow heartbeat or
reduce the contraction of the heart. This is an important cause of
low blood pressure. Patients with severe heart failure may present
with signs and symptoms of poor blood flow due to their low
blood pressure. This is known as cardiogenic shock and is a life-
threatening condition requiring urgent treatment to improve heart
function. A common cause of cardiogenic shock is severe damage to
the heart caused by a heart attack. Emergency hospital treatment to
improve blood flow to the heart can be life-saving.

Other causes of low blood pressure include bleeding and dehydra-
tion. These conditions lead to a reduction in the circulating blood
volume (hypovolaemic shock). Severe infection (septic shock) can
also cause low blood pressure due to release of toxins and low vascular resistance. Acutely sick patients with low blood pressure are
often treated in hospital intensive care units. These patients need

to be carefully monitored and treated with intravenous fluids and drugs to increase vascular resistance. This will increase their blood pressure to acceptable levels, which will prevent organ damage caused by inadequate blood flow.

Systolic and diastolic blood pressure

Our blood pressure is made up of two components: a peak and a trough. The peak – systolic – blood pressure is generated by the contraction (systole) of the heart, during which blood is forcefully ejected from the heart. The trough – diastolic pressure – occurs when the heart relaxes (diastole) and blood pressure falls as the heart starts filling with blood. Blood pressure is measured in millimetres of mercury (mmHg). The systolic blood pressure is recorded first and then the diastolic pressure. Someone with a systolic blood pressure of 140 mmHg and diastolic blood pressure of 80 mmHg would be told that his or her blood pressure was 140 over 80, which is written as 140/80. Diastolic blood pressure does not fall rapidly between heartbeats because of the elasticity of the arteries. Some of the force generated by each heart contraction is stored as energy in the arteries as they stretch (this is known as the elastic reservoir capacity). This force is released during diastole to maintain pressure in the circulation. You can imagine this if you think of the air trapped in a blown-up balloon; the trapped air is under pressure due to the elastic forces stored in the balloon wall. The arteries act as pressure reservoirs that constantly absorb and release elastic force to maintain the pressure in the circulation.

What is pulse pressure?

The difference between systolic and diastolic blood pressure readings is known as the pulse pressure. As people get older the large arteries in the body become progressively stiffer. This causes an increase in systolic blood pressure, a decrease in diastolic blood pressure and a widening of the pulse pressure. A pulse pressure of more than approximately 55 mmHg in people aged over 60 is another risk factor for heart disease, because it often reflects an increased arterial stiffness caused by fatty deposits in the arterial wall. Another cause for a wide pulse pressure is damage to the aortic valve, which is the main heart valve that opens to let blood leave the heart during each heart contraction. During relaxation, or diastole, of the heart, the aortic valve closes to prevent blood leaking back into the heart. A faulty valve does not completely shut during diastole allowing blood to regurgitate back from the aorta to fill the heart. One of the signs of severe aortic valve incompetence is a wide pulse pressure.

Regulation of blood pressure

Baroreceptors and the autonomic nervous system

The body has a complex system for monitoring its own blood pressure. This system is continuously adapting to our physiological requirements to ensure that our blood pressure is maintained within a normal range. Specialised pressure sensors called baroreceptors are present in the aortic arch and carotid sinuses. These areas are richly innervated with nerve endings that respond to the stretching of the arterial wall during each heartbeat. The nerve inputs conduct signals back to the blood pressure-regulating centre located in the brain stem. This is the stem-like section of the brain that connects the brain hemispheres to the spinal cord, and, in evolutionary terms, is thought to be the oldest part of the brain. If the blood pressure rises suddenly, signals are sent from the baroreceptors to the brainstem, which acts to decrease blood pressure using the autonomic nervous system.

The two main systems used by the body for blood pressure balance are the autonomic system and the kidneys. Historically, hypertension research focused on how the kidneys control blood pressure. However, recent work to develop new hypertension treatments has increased the attention given to the role of the autonomic system. The autonomic nervous system comprises a complex network of nerves throughout the body that consists of the sympathetic nervous system and the parasympathetic nervous system. These two parts work in opposite ways, like yin and yang, to maintain balance (homeostasis) in the body. The sympathetic system prepares the body for action and increases blood pressure by increasing our heart rate, force of heart contractions and vascular resistance. Exercise and stress activate the sympathetic system and lead to increases in blood pressure. This means that it is important to have your blood pressure measured when you are sitting down and relaxed, with a resting heart rate that is typically between 60 and 100 beats per minute. If you have been rushed to the clinic, you must make sure that you are seated and comfortable before having a blood pressure reading. The parasympathetic system relaxes the body and decreases blood pressure by slowing the heart rate, reducing the force of heart contractions and lowering the vascular resistance. The baroreceptor system is excellent at adapting to sudden changes in blood pressure. It is very responsive and works in minutes. However, it is not as effective for persistent elevation in blood pressure, which is thought to be often caused by chronic over-activation of the sympathetic system.

Blood pressure control and the kidneys

The kidneys receive a significant portion of the blood flow during each heartbeat. As well as filtering the blood, the kidneys contain numerous specialised cells that monitor blood pressure. If blood pressure falls, the kidneys sense this as a reduced blood flow and activate the RAAS (renin–angiotensin–aldosterone) system. Cells in the kidneys release a chemical messenger (hormone) called renin. This acts via angiotensin II (which is a hormone produced by the liver) to stimulate the release of aldosterone from the adrenal glands. Aldosterone is a potent hormone that increases blood pressure by causing constriction in blood vessels. Aldosterone also promotes salt retention by the kidneys, leading to higher salt, or sodium, levels that cause an increased blood volume and elevation in blood pressure.

The RAAS system is the target of several classes of drugs used to treat high blood pressure. These drugs include angiotensin converting enzyme (ACE) inhibitors, angiotensin receptor blockers (ARBS) and aldosterone receptor blockers. The RAAS system acts more slowly than the baroreceptors and causes a more persistent elevation in blood pressure. Chronically high blood pressure is often caused by abnormalities of kidney function along with activation of the RAAS system.

Diurnal variation in blood pressure

Blood pressure varies throughout the day, following a daily pattern that gives higher readings in the morning and lower readings in the evening. Your blood pressure starts to rise a few hours after you wake up and continues to rise during the day, peaking at mid-afternoon, and at its lowest during the evenings and at night. The typical variation in blood pressure can be between 10–15 mmHg for the systolic pressure and 5–10 mmHg for diastolic pressure. Therefore, if your blood pressure is 150/90 mmHg in the afternoon it may be as low as 135/80 mmHg during the night.

In healthy people, sleep reduces both systolic and diastolic blood pressure by 10–15 per cent, which is known as nocturnal blood pressure dipping. This is caused by changes in the balance of the autonomic nervous system, with reductions in sympathetic drive and the predominance of parasympathetic activity. This sleep-related blood pressure dipping is important for normal cardio-vascular health, and if it doesn't happen, there is an increased risk of heart disease. Obstructive sleep apnoea, an intermittent obstruction to normal breathing (see Chapter 4), is a common cause of both daytime and nocturnal hypertension because of the frequent interruptions in breathing.

It is important to remember this normal diurnal variation in blood pressure when diagnosing hypertension, as this diagnosis is often made on the basis of a reading during the afternoon blood pressure peak. Diagnosing hypertension can be done more accurately when blood pressure levels are monitored throughout the day (see Chapter 4) and the calculation of average blood pressure, ideally, should be based on several readings.

2
How do you measure blood pressure?

A brief history of blood pressure measurements

Pressure is a force which was originally measured by its ability to displace a column of liquid using a device called a manometer. Most liquid manometers use mercury, as its high density allows the use of a shorter column to measure a given pressure. In 1773, the English scientist Stephen Hales recorded the first blood pressure measurement by connecting a series of glass tubes to the artery of a horse. He showed that the column of blood rose in the tube eight feet above the level of the heart and rose and fell with each of the horse's heartbeats.

The first non-invasive blood pressure measurement was performed in 1896 by the Italian physician Riva-Rocci. He described the method that is similar to the modern system of blood pressure recording. Riva-Rocci used a cuff which is inflated and thus compresses the arm, just above the elbow. As the cuff is inflated, a point is reached when the pressure in the cuff is high enough to overcome systolic pressure and block the blood flow in the brachial artery in the arm. As the cuff is deflated, systolic pressure is recorded at the cuff pressure when the pulse is first felt. This method is still used today for rapid assessment of systolic pressure, but it cannot measure diastolic pressure.

Measuring systolic and diastolic blood pressure

In 1905 the Russian physician Dr Korotkoff invented the auscultatory, or sound technique, for measuring blood pressure. This method can measure both systolic and diastolic blood pressure and is the standard technique still used today. To measure blood pressure, a cuff is inflated across the upper arm to compress the main artery (brachial artery). The cuff is then slowly deflated, and

14

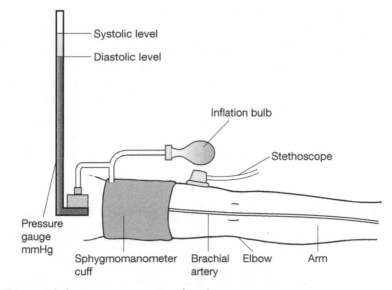

Figure 4 Sphygmomanometer showing pressure gauge

the person taking the measurement monitors the cuff pressure and uses a stethoscope to listen to the brachial artery just above the elbow. The systolic blood pressure is recorded when the first sounds of blood flowing past the cuff is heard. The diastolic blood pressure measurement is taken when the sound just disappears. Originally, mercury sphygmomanometers were used to measure blood pressure, so by convention, blood pressure is still recorded in millimetres of mercury (mmHg) (Figure 4).

Mercury sphygmomanometers have now been replaced with aneroid (liquid-free) devices that use a moving pointer on a circular scale to document pressure. If you have your blood pressure checked by your GP, they are likely to use an aneroid sphygmomanometer. Automatic sphygmomanometers use a digital display and pressure sensors that document the blood pressure as the cuff slowly deflates; these digital readings are converted and displayed as mmHg. Although automated blood pressure recordings are accurate, the auscultatory method is considered as the gold standard for recording blood pressure, so automated blood pressure devices need to be validated, and regularly maintained and calibrated according to the manufacturer's instructions.

Automated blood pressure devices may not give an accurate reading in patients with an irregular pulse (for example, in patients with atrial fibrillation). These patients should have their blood pressure measured manually using the auscultation method. The British Hypertension Society website (<www.bhsoc.org>) has a list of validated blood pressure monitoring devices that are currently available. Wrist blood pressure devices are not recommended for recording blood pressure to use for a diagnosis of hypertension as these measurements do not compare with readings made from the upper arm.

How to take an accurate blood pressure recording

This procedure should be followed to obtain an accurate blood pressure measurement in the clinic.

- The cuff should fit snugly, with a size appropriate to your build – larger cuffs for patients with wide arms and smaller cuffs for patients with thinner arms. If the cuff is too small for your arm, the blood pressure measurement will appear higher than it really is.
- You should be relaxed and have been seated for around 3–5 minutes before having your blood pressure taken.
- Your arm should be at the level of your heart (mid-chest).
- Two blood pressure measurements should be made one to two minutes apart.
- On your first visit to the clinic, the pressure in both arms should be checked. A significant difference between these measurements (that is, more than 20 mmHg) could indicate a narrowing of the subclavian or axillary artery in your upper arm on the side with the lower reading. For the purposes of monitoring, always record the blood pressure in the arm with the higher reading during subsequent checks.

Ambulatory blood pressure monitoring

Your blood pressure changes constantly, depending upon the time of day, your posture, emotional state and how much exercise you have done. Also, blood pressure readings tend to be higher in the afternoon and lower at night, which means that it is difficult to make decisions on whether to initiate treatment for hypertension based on a single set, or even a few sets, of blood pressure readings. In true hypertension, blood pressure is persistently elevated throughout the day. One method used to assess blood pressure profiles during the day is 24-hour ambulatory blood pressure (AMBP) recording.

AMBP devices are easy to fit, and consist of a small portable digital blood pressure machine that is attached to a belt strapped around the waist. The monitor is connected to a cuff wrapped around the upper arm (Figure 5).

You wear the device during normal activity at home, and, typically, blood pressure is recorded twice every hour during the day and once an hour during the night. You are usually instructed to maintain your normal routine, but to avoid strenuous exercise. Walking around with a cuff attached to the arm can be difficult

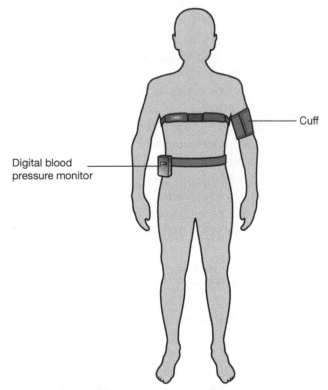

Cuff

Digital blood
pressure monitor

Figure 5 Ambulatory blood pressure monitor

Table 2 Normal blood pressure measured with an ambulatory blood pressure recorder

Daytime	mmHg
Normal systolic	≤ 135
Normal diastolic	≤ 85
Night time	
Normal systolic	≤ 120
Normal diastolic	≤ 70

and many people find having the monitor on during the night very intrusive. However, this monitoring does provide a comprehensive and consistent view of what is actually going on with your blood pressure, and avoids the problem of 'white coat hypertension' (see Chapter 4). The data is downloaded onto a computer, and software is used to produce a graphical display of blood pressure readings during the recording period. At least 14 readings during a day are required for the data to be valid and the data is summarised as the average systolic and diastolic blood pressure during the day and night (Table 2).

AMBP measurements are better at predicting the development of organ damage and adverse cardiovascular events than blood pressure readings taken in GP surgeries. This monitoring provides a real-life profile of blood pressure away from the medical environment. Multiple blood pressure readings at home are more reflective of true blood pressure and a significant proportion of people whose blood pressure shows a mild elevation at their GPs will have normal AMBP readings. For these people, wearing the AMBP device is worth the discomfort, as it means that they won't need lifelong drug treatment for hypertension.

In the UK, the National Institute for Health and Care Excellence (NICE) has published guidelines that have brought ABPM into much wider clinical use. NICE has recommended that ABPM, or home blood pressure monitoring, is used to confirm the diagnosis of hypertension in all those with mild to moderate elevation in blood pressure before drug treatment is started. ABPM is now available in many GP surgeries that have the appropriate software to produce accurate results. ABPM is useful for:

- people with suspected white coat hypertension (that is, people who have high blood pressure readings and no signs of organ damage);
- people who have very variable blood pressure readings;
- the confirmation of a diagnosis in people with mild elevation in blood pressure readings;
- people who have persistent elevation in blood pressure despite taking several medications;
- monitoring the response to treatment.

Home blood pressure monitoring

The home blood pressure monitoring (HBPM) technique is used to self-monitor blood pressure at home using a personal automated digital blood pressure machine. For each blood pressure reading,

Table 3 Suggested template for recording your blood pressure measurements taken at home

Date	Time	Systolic blood pressure	Diastolic blood pressure	Pulse rate
Day 1	a.m.			
	p.m.			
Day 2	a.m.			
	p.m.			
Day 3	a.m.			
	p.m.			
Day 4	a.m.			
	p.m.			
Day 5	a.m.			
	p.m.			
Day 6	a.m.			
	p.m.			
Day 7	a.m.			
	p.m.			
Average blood pressure				

take two consecutive measurements at least one to two minutes apart. Sit with your back and arm supported and take the measurements after five minutes' rest. Don't use the measurements taken on the first day, but calculate the average value of all the remaining measurements to give you your home blood pressure. You should measure your blood pressure on at least five (and preferably seven) consecutive days, taking readings in the morning and evening. Table 3 gives a template that you could use to record your blood pressure.

HBPM is better at predicting cardiovascular morbidity and mortality than blood pressure readings done at GP surgeries, and this prognostic significance is similar to that of ABPM. People find that HBPM is easier and less intrusive than ABPM, and it is not as costly. It increases people's sense of involvement and empowerment in the management of their conditions, which makes them more motivated to stick to lifestyle changes and take the medications as prescribed. However, unlike ABPM, home monitoring does not provide data during normal routine daytime activities and when sleeping, so it is not suitable for everyone. NICE recommends that both ABPM and HBPM can be used to confirm a diagnosis of hypertension.

Central blood pressure

Central blood pressure is measured close to the heart from the aorta, the main artery that carries blood from the heart to the rest of the body. These measurements tend to be lower than traditional blood pressure readings taken from the brachial artery in the upper arm. As the blood pressure wave travels away from the heart, the systolic peak pressure is amplified due to increasing arterial stiffness; diastolic pressures remain unchanged. Central blood pressure may be better than brachial blood pressure for predicting the risk of complications of high blood pressure, as the major organs that are damaged by high blood pressure (that is, the heart, brain and kidneys) are exposed to central blood pressure rather than brachial blood pressure. Drugs have different abilities to lower central blood pressure, with beta blockers having a reduced ability to lower central blood pressure than some other drugs.

The importance of central blood pressure was shown in a major trial examining high blood pressure called the Anglo Scandinavian

Cardiac Outcomes Trial (ASCOT). The principal finding of this large study, which involved more than 19,000 patients, was that amlodipine-based blood-pressure lowering treatments were superior in preventing stroke and death compared to the beta blocker atenolol.[2] Another study carried out using data from the ASCOT trial showed that amlodipine was superior to atenolol in lowering central blood pressure, whereas there were similar reductions in brachial blood pressure in the two groups.[3] This indicates that lowering central blood pressure is the main factor that determines cardiovascular protection. However, at present, central blood pressure measurements are only used for research and have not replaced brachial blood pressure measurements in clinical practice. This is due both to the ease of measuring brachial blood pressure and to the lack of guidance as to what level of central blood pressure needs treatment. Non-invasive techniques to measure central blood pressure use probes with pressure sensors that record the arterial waveforms from the arteries in the neck. In the future, central blood pressure monitoring may replace traditional cuff-based brachial pressure checks.

3

Risks associated with high blood pressure

There are still many people with high blood pressure who remain unaware of its risks, despite the alarming statistics on its effects on health, increased awareness of the condition and the availability of regular routine monitoring. Being aware of the dangers of high blood pressure is helpful in spurring people on to make essential lifestyle adjustments or to take the prescribed medication, without which the doctor's efforts are in vain. Don't let a stroke or other cardiovascular event be your first warning of the risks of high blood pressure! Arm yourself with knowledge so that you understand which measures to take to improve your future. In the USA it is estimated that around 1,000 deaths a day are due to high blood pressure. Hypertension is present in:

- seven out of ten people who have their first heart attack;
- eight out of ten people who have their first stroke;
- seven out of ten people with chronic heart failure.

High blood pressure exerts excessive strain on the cardiovascular system, involving four body systems: the heart, arteries, brain and kidneys. It increases the risk of death from stroke four-fold and from heart disease three-fold. For every 20/10 mmHg increase in blood pressure, the risk of cardiovascular disease doubles. Conversely, even small reductions in blood pressure can have significant and positive impacts on health, so do not be discouraged to take action. Reducing a high diastolic blood pressure by 6 mmHg is estimated to reduce the risk of stroke by 35–40 per cent and the risk of cardio-vascular disease by 20–25 per cent. Larger reductions provide even greater benefits.

Effects of high blood pressure on the heart

The effects of high blood pressure on the heart include:

- thickening of the heart muscle (left ventricular hypertrophy) (Figure 6);
- heart failure, involving shortness of breath and fluid congestion;
- atrial fibrillation (a rapid and irregular heart beat), which is a major cause of stroke.

It is useful to think of blood pressure as a force, as it helps to understand the consequences of hypertension and reasons for organ damage. Increased vascular resistance causes most cases of high blood pressure. To maintain an adequate blood supply to the tissues, the heart has to work harder at pumping blood against increased resistance. The long-term effects of high blood pressure on the heart are increased thickening of the heart muscle (hypertrophy) and scarring (fibrosis). As the heart muscle becomes thicker and more scarred, its ability to relax and fill with blood between contractions is impaired. The net effect of these changes is that the pressure in the left side of the heart rises, which leads to the signs and symptoms of heart failure known as diastolic heart failure.

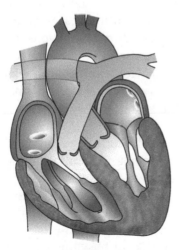
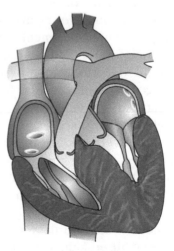

Normal heart   Hypertrophic heart

Figure 6 Left ventricular hypertrophy

This contrasts to systolic heart failure in which the main problem is a weakness of contraction and pump failure. Approximately half of all patients with heart failure, especially elderly patients, will have diastolic heart failure. High pressure in the heart is transmitted back to the lungs and the venous circulation and people with heart failure often complain of swollen legs and shortness of breath, due to fluid in the lungs and lower limbs. This can be very debilitating and people may need 'water' tablets (diuretics) to remove the excessive fluid to alleviate the swelling in the legs and breathlessness.

Hypertension can also cause scarring and stretching of the atria – the small chambers at the back of the heart. This leads to a common rhythm problem of the heart called atrial fibrillation, in which the heartbeat is very fast and irregular. While there are many causes of atrial fibrillation, in Europe and the USA hypertension is the most common cause, particularly in the elderly. The most serious complication of atrial fibrillation is if a clot forms in the atria. If the clot dislodges, it can block arteries in the brain, for example, leading to brain damage and stroke. If you have both hypertension and atrial fibrillation, your doctor should consider you for long-term treatment with blood thinners (anticoagulants) to prevent stroke. Until recently, warfarin was the only available anticoagulant and many people are reluctant to take warfarin, due to the need for regular blood tests to monitor treatment and frequent dose adjustments, and its multiple drug interactions. For example, you should not routinely take aspirin or ibuprofen if you are on warfarin. Warfarin also interacts with alcohol and some foods and drinks, such as foods high in vitamin K (for example, green leafy vegetables, such as spinach and broccoli) and cranberry and grapefruit juice.

Over the last two years, however, new oral anticoagulants have provided an alternative to warfarin for people with atrial fibrillation. Drugs such as dabigatran, rivaroxaban and apixaban are as effective, or better, than warfarin at preventing stroke (and are associated with fewer bleeding complications). Blood test monitoring is not needed and daily fixed doses are taken. The dose taken is dependent on kidney function and any risks of bleeding. GPs will also provide information regarding any drug interactions with any other medication taken. If you are on new oral anticogulants, it is important to inform your health or dental professional before any procedure. All the new oral anticoagulants have a lower rate of bleeding into the brain (intracranial haemorrhage) compared to warfarin (an average of 0.4 per cent per year compared to 0.8 per cent per year with warfarin).

Effects of high blood pressure on the arteries

The effects of high blood pressure on the arteries include:

- hardening of the arteries (atherosclerosis), causing angina and heart attacks;
- weakness of major arteries, leading to aneurysm formation and risk of rupture;
- the possibility of a tear (dissection) in the lining of the aorta (the main artery);
- possible damage to the blood vessels in the back of the eye (retina).

Atherosclerosis is caused by inflammation of the inner lining of the arteries and deposition of fatty material (atheroma) as plaques (Figure 7).

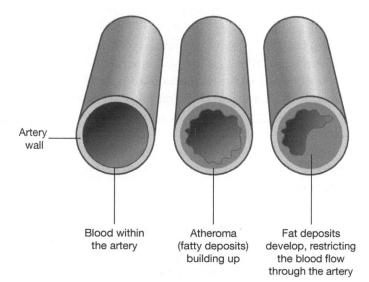

Artery wall

Blood within the artery

Atheroma (fatty deposits) building up

Fat deposits develop, restricting the blood flow through the artery

Figure 7 How atheroma develops

Atherosclerosis in the heart arteries reduces the diameter of the arteries and obstructs blood flow; this is known as ischaemic heart disease. This causes chest tightness on exertion (angina), and can cause heart attack and sudden death. Ischaemic heart disease is also the leading cause of heart failure due to reduced pump function (systolic heart failure). Atherosclerosis in the arteries of the lower limbs can cause the signs and symptoms of poor blood flow. You can develop cramp in the back of the calves on exertion (intermittent claudication) and, in severe cases, pain in fingers or toes, and even tissue death (necrosis).

The aorta is the main artery that carries blood from the heart to the rest of the body. Patients with hypertension are at risk of excessive outward stretching of the aorta, with atherosclerosis leading to localised weakening of the vessel wall, so that it bulges outwards to form an aneurysm. Aneurysms of the aorta in the chest or abdomen can rupture, which is a life-threatening complication needing emergency surgical treatment. In the UK, abdominal aortic aneurysm (AAA) screening is being introduced for all men aged 65 years or over. This involves having an ultrasound scan of the abdomen, which is a non-invasive scan that takes 10–15 minutes to perform. The normal diameter of the abdominal aorta is around 2 cm, but sometimes this blood vessel can distend further. If that is the case, then more frequent ultrasound scans will be needed to keep an eye on its size. Uncontrolled hypertension can weaken the lining of the aorta, making it more prone to tearing. Aortic dissection is a medical emergency when a tear in the aortic wall spirals down the aorta leading to bleeding into the arterial wall. If this happens, the symptoms are acute severe chest or back pain, and patients often collapse. Urgent early diagnosis and treatment are required. Patients often have a history of hypertension, and blood pressure can be high on admission. Intensive blood pressure control is required in patients who do not need immediate surgery.

Effects of high blood pressure on the brain

Our awareness of the impact of high blood pressure on the brain is growing. Several studies have looked at the link between raised blood pressure and increased risk of dementia, and, more generally, it is accepted that 'what's good for the heart is good for the brain'. Keeping blood pressure under control and exercising regularly help prevent dementia.

The main risks of high blood pressure on the brain are:

- ischaemic and haemorrhagic stroke
- multi-infarct dementia
- cognitive impairment.

Hypertension is a major risk factor for acute brain injury due to stroke. In Europe and the USA, stroke is the third most common cause of death, after heart disease and cancer. Yet stroke is preventable, and reducing your blood pressure is key to its prevention. Sadly, those most likely to take preventative action are those who have already had a stroke, although the good news here is that a further stroke can be prevented in up to 80 per cent of cases. Take heed, especially if you have a family history of stroke.

There are two types of stroke: ischaemic and haemorrhagic. High blood pressure increases the risk of both types of stroke, particularly haemorrhagic stroke. Ischaemic stroke accounts for 90 per cent of all strokes and is caused by the sudden blockage of a brain artery due to a clot leading to ischaemic (lack of blood) brain damage. Symptoms may be mild or severe and many people do not survive the first stroke. Hypertension causes deposition of fatty plaques in the walls of the arteries, which can break away from the vessel wall and travel down the circulation to occlude small vessels in the brain. Hypertension can also cause atrial fibrillation, which is responsible for around 25 per cent of all ischaemic strokes. Haemorrhagic stroke is caused by bleeding into the brain; it is usually severe and often fatal. High blood pressure in the small vessels deep in the brain causes weakness and increased risk of rupture.

Dementia is a group of conditions in which there is progressive decline in brain function, often causing memory loss. Alzheimer's disease is the most common cause of dementia. Multiple strokes can cause a stepwise deterioration in brain function leading to a type of dementia known as multi-infarct dementia. People who have high blood pressure in middle age have a greater decline in brain function over the following 20 years than people with normal blood pressure. Treatment of blood pressure with medication can help prevent deterioration in cognitive ability and reduce stroke risks.

Effects of high blood pressure on the kidneys

Narrowing of the blood vessels in the kidneys can lead to kidney failure, tell-tale signs of which are protein or blood in the urine. The kidneys are intricately involved in the regulation of blood volume because they control the amount of fluid retained in the blood versus the amount lost as waste in the urine. High blood pressure can damage the small blood vessels in the kidneys, making them unable to filter waste from the blood (in the form of urine). The National Heart, Lung, and Blood Institute, one of the US National Institutes of Health, recommends that people with diabetes or impaired kidney function keep their blood pressure below 140/90,[4] which is a change from the 2003 guidelines that suggested a target blood pressure of below 130/80.[5]

The effects of high blood pressure on the kidneys are:

- kidney failure with a decline in filtration rate and protein in the urine;
- further increase in blood pressure due to the salt and water retention caused by the kidney damage.

The main function of the kidneys is to filter waste products and excessive water from the blood; these are excreted from the body as urine. Just over one litre of blood passes through the kidneys each minute, with around 10 per cent being filtered. Each kidney contains around 1 million individual units called nephrons. Each nephron contains a bundle of tiny blood vessels, called glomeruli, that work like a sieve. As blood is pushed through the glomeruli, water and waste products are removed, while nutrients and important proteins are retained. High blood pressure causes excessive stretching and scarring of the tiny blood vessels forming the glomeruli. Damaged glomeruli are unable to filter blood effectively, leading to a decline in the filtration rate and presence of abnormal amounts of protein in the blood. There are a limited number of kidney nephrons in your body, and once damaged these cannot be regenerated.

Table 4 Five stages of kidney disease

Stage	Description	Glomerular filtration rate (GFR)
1	Kidney damage (proteinuria) with normal GFR	90 or above
2	Mild decline in kidney function	60–89
3	Moderate decline in kidney function	30–59
4	Severe decline in kidney function	15–29
5	End-stage kidney failure	Less than 15

The kidney plays an important role in the regulation of blood pressure, through the control of blood volume and salt levels. The kidney also produces hormones that cause vasoconstriction and increase vascular resistance. Over time, any cause of kidney damage increases blood pressure because of the accumulation of salt and extra fluid. The prevalence of hypertension is around 20 per cent in people with mild chronic kidney disease and 80 per cent in people with severe chronic kidney disease.

Treating high blood pressure has been shown to prevent kidney disease from getting worse and to reduce protein levels in the urine. There are two ways of detecting kidney damage:

1 A blood test that measures waste product (creatinine) levels, which is used to estimate the glomerular filtration rate (GFR). As kidney disease progresses, the GFR number declines and creatinine levels increase (Table 4).
2 A urine test for blood and protein. This quick test uses a urine dipstick that changes colour if blood or protein is detected.

Effects of high blood pressure on the eyes

Sustained high blood pressure can damage the small blood vessels in the back of the eye that supply the retina. This is the part of the eye that contains the specialised light-sensitive cells onto which light is focused, enabling vision. You may have noticed that your optometrist often comments on your health during routine eye examinations. This is because looking at the retina provides a window to examine the circulation, as the retinal arteries share similar properties to arteries in the heart and brain. The most common eye sign of high blood pressure is thickening of the retinal arteries, which is seen as a change in the normal light reflex when examined with a slit lamp or ophthalmoscope. In more advanced disease stages, additional changes include retinal bleeds (haemorrhages), small dilated sections of blood vessels (aneurysms) and tissue swelling (oedema). Symptoms can include headaches and vision disturbance.

4

Diagnosing hypertension

All patients with high blood pressure should be fully evaluated: this should include taking a medical history, doing a physical examination, running blood tests, doing a urine analysis, heart electrical tracing (electrocardiogram) and, possibly, carrying out an ultrasound scan of the heart (echocardiogram). This type of thorough examination looks for additional risk factors as well as high blood pressure, and any evidence of organ damage and should pick up any possible secondary causes of hypertension.

Medical history

Your doctor should check for additional cardiovascular risk factors such as diabetes, smoking, and a family history of premature cardiac disease or hypertension. You are more likely to be started on treatment earlier if you are considered to have multiple risk factors for hypertension. Ideally, the treatment prescribed should be holistic and address all risk factors, rather that just aiming for better blood pressure control.

Family history is a significant risk factor in high blood pressure. A positive family history is having a first-degree family member who was diagnosed with hypertension or had a heart attack before the age of 60. A significant number of people with high blood pressure have a strong family history of hypertension, suggesting an underlying genetic cause. Hypertension is about twice as common in people who have one or two hypertensive parents. The genetics of hypertension is complex and single gene mutations causing elevation in blood pressure are rare. This means that genetic testing is not a useful tool, as multiple genes contribute to the development of hypertension. The medications that you are taking should be reviewed, as several treatments can increase blood pressure (see Chapter 5). Excessive alcohol intake and a high-salt diet are known to contribute to hypertension and correcting these is a priority (see Chapter 9).

Symptoms of chest tightness or breathlessness on exertion should be screened for, as these may point to an underlying heart disease. Any past medical history of heart disease or stroke suggests the need for blood pressure better control. Another common cause of blood pressure elevation is interrupted breathing during sleep (obstructive sleep apnoea), which has troublesome symptoms such as poor concentration, daytime sleepiness, and snoring. If this is suspected, you should be referred for specialist sleep studies, as obstructive sleep apnoea is treatable.

Physical examination

Your doctor will want to check whether your high blood pressure has affected any part of your body, and will take your general health into account when assessing this. For example, obesity is a common cause of high blood pressure and your doctor may want to measure your height, weight and body mass index (BMI). Your general appearance can sometimes offer other clues of underlying endocrine abnormalities that can cause high blood pressure, such as thyroid disease, acromegaly and Cushing's disease. Bulbous eyes are a well-known sign of an overactive thyroid (hyperthyroidism), for example, but your doctor will also be alert for more subtle signs of illness, such as thinning or missing eyebrows, or rough, dry skin caused by an underactive thyroid (hypothyroidism), or the typical moon face of Cushing's syndrome, caused by high levels of the hormone cortisol.

Your doctor will want to check for signs of heart failure, including swelling of the neck veins and ankles, and hearing crackles in the chest. He or she may also listen to your heart with a stethoscope, which could reveal additional heart sounds (murmurs) suggesting abnormal function of the heart valves. In this case, you may be referred for a special ultrasound scan of the heart, known as an echocardiogram, which will look in detail at the structural aspects of the heart. Your doctor may also test the pulse in your groin. Absent or weak pulses here may suggest a congenital narrowing of the aorta (coarctation) as the cause of hypertension. This is more common in young male patients. Your doctor may also want to examine your eyes. As explained above, severe hypertension can cause changes in the blood vessels at the back of the eye, and your doctor may use an ophthalmoscope to examine the retina.

Blood tests

When you are diagnosed with high blood pressure, your doctor or nurse may carry out routine blood tests to check how well your body is coping, and to help plan your treatment. Routine blood tests include tests for:

- anaemia;
- kidney function;
- diabetes;
- cholesterol levels;
- low blood potassium levels;
- excluding the possibility of thyroid disease.

If you have hypertension and ischaemic heart disease, you will need to take a statin to lower cholesterol levels and reduce the risk of a heart attack. If you have high blood pressure and low blood potassium levels, you may need additional blood tests to look for a rare endocrine disorder of the adrenal glands called Conn's syndrome, which causes the excess production of a hormone called aldosterone.

Urine analysis

A urine test with a dipstick is swift, painless and useful. It will detect any blood or protein in the urine, which can be a sign of chronic kidney disease (see Chapter 3). A simple urine test can be performed rapidly at the GP surgery, using indicator sticks that change colour when exposed to protein or blood in the urine. The colour change can be read off a scale to quantify the amount of protein or blood present. Sometimes your doctor will need more information, in which case a more detailed assessment is obtained by sending a urine sample to the laboratory to measure protein levels. Occasionally, 24-hour urine collection in special containers is required to calculate kidney function. The urine will be assessed for protein excretion and used to measure hormone levels.

Electrocardiogram

An electrocardiogram, or ECG, records your heart rhythm. This non-invasive procedure detects the electrical activity of the heart muscle and shows an electrical tracing of the heart. Patients with hypertension are more likely to develop an irregular heart rhythm (such as atrial fibrillation), which is detected on the ECG. Long-standing high blood pressure can cause thickening of the heart muscle (hypertrophy), which can also cause high voltages on the ECG. In addition, an ECG can show signs of a previous heart attack, due to changes in electrical conduction, which indicate underlying structural heart disease.

Echocardiogram

This is an ultrasound examination of the heart, taken through the chest, in which sound waves transmit images to a video monitor. This is a useful test that looks for structural heart disease. If the ECG is abnormal, or there are signs of heart disease, an echocardiogram is often performed. The echocardiogram is more accurate than an ECG at detecting hypertrophy. It can also assess the function of the heart valves, look at the force of heart contractions, and measure the size of the heart chambers. High blood pressure can cause dilatation of the main artery arising from the heart (ascending aorta) and incompetence of the aortic valve. Both of these conditions can be detected by an echocardiogram.

Cardiac magnetic resonance imaging

Hypertension specialists may refer some patients with high blood pressure for a cardiac magnetic resonance imaging (MRI) scan, in which the patient lies inside a large circular magnetic scanner. The scan may last for up to an hour. The magnetic field causes the cells in the body to emit radiation waves, which are detected by the scanner to produce images of the heart. Cardiac MRI scans can show secondary causes of hypertension, such as narrowing of the kidney arteries, congenital narrowing of the aorta, kidney cysts or tumours of the adrenal glands. The cardiac MRI also enables the recording of precise measurements of the strength of heart contractions, thickness of heart muscle and chamber size.

Organ damage

Everyone with hypertension should be carefully screened for asymptomatic organ damage – that is, damage that you may not be aware of – and established cardiovascular or renal disease. Asymptomatic organ damage can be diagnosed as described below.

- Thickening of the heart muscle (left ventricular hypertrophy) seen on the ECG or echocardiogram.
- A wide pulse pressure (more than 60 mmHg difference in systolic and diastolic blood pressure) in the elderly.
- An ankle brachial pressure index (ABPI) of less than 0.9 in patients with impaired circulation in the legs. ABPI is a test used to diagnose significant narrowing of the arteries in the lower limbs (peripheral vascular disease). In healthy people the systolic pressure in the ankle is the same as the systolic pressure in the arm. The ABPI is the ratio between these two systolic blood pressures. An ABPI of less than 0.9 indicates significant peripheral vascular disease.
- Having a blood test showing moderate chronic kidney disease with estimated glomerular filtration rates (eGFR) of 30–60 mL/min/1.73 m^2 (the normal eGFR is $\geq$90 mL/min/1.73 m^2).
- Having significant protein in the urine. This can be tested by urine dip stick, spot urine analysis or 24-hour urine collection. Microalbuminuria (small amounts of protein) is defined as 30–300 mg protein per 24 hours or a morning spot sample of urine with an albumen:creatinine ratio of >2.5 mg/mmol (for men) and >3.5 mg/mmol (for women). An albumen:creatinine ratio of >30 mg/mmol is defined as significant proteinuria and is no longer in the range for microalbuminuria.

Established cardiovascular or renal disease includes having:

- coronary artery disease with angina, a previous heart attack, a history of coronary angioplasty and stents or coronary artery bypass surgery;
- heart failure;
- cerebrovascular disease (stroke or transient ischaemic attack or brain haemorrhage);
- symptomatic peripheral vascular disease;

- chronic kidney disease with an eGFR of less than 30 mL/ min/1.73 m² or severe protein loss in the urine (that is, more than 300 mg per 24 hours);
- significant damage to the retina with retinal bleeds or leaking of protein.

Definition of hypertension

For practical reasons a single threshold is used above which the diagnosis of hypertension is made. This level is based on the results of clinical trials that have shown the benefits of blood-pressure lowering treatment. There is general agreement that people with sustained readings of systolic blood pressure equal to or higher than (≥) 140 and/or diastolic pressure ≥90 have hypertension. This value is used in all adults irrespective of age and gender. However, in young children and adolescents there is no single cut-off at which hypertension is diagnosed and high blood pressure is defined according to normal values found in that age group. Both systolic and diastolic readings are important and hypertension is diagnosed if the diastolic reading is high even when the systolic is below 140 mmHg.

Grading of hypertension

There are three grades of hypertension that are based either on clinic, ambulatory or home blood pressure readings. Stage 1 is mild hypertension with a clinic blood pressure ≥140 systolic and/or a diastolic pressure ≥90 mmHg. On home or AMBP monitoring stage 1 hypertension corresponds to an average daytime systolic pressure ≥135 and/or diastolic ≥85 mmHg. Stage 2 hypertension is diagnosed when the clinic systolic blood pressure is ≥160 and/or diastolic is ≥100 mmHg. Stage 3, or severe hypertension, is diagnosed when systolic blood pressure is ≥180 and/or diastolic ≥ 110 mmHg. Some national guidelines have now incorporated stage 3 hypertension in with stage 2. However, some clinicians still refer to stage 3, or severe hypertension, for patients with blood pressure of more than 180/110 mmHg.

Isolated systolic hypertension is found mainly in those over the age of 65, with elevated systolic blood pressure (140 mmHg) and normal diastolic blood pressure (less than 90 mmHg) (Table 5).

Table 5 Stages of hypertension

Definition of hypertension stages	Clinic blood pressure	Ambulatory or home blood pressure (daytime average)
Not hypertensive	< 140/90	< 135/85
Stage 1	≥ 140/90	≥ 135/85
Stage 2	≥ 160/100	≥ 150/95
Stage 3 – severe	≥ 180/110	
Isolated systolic hypertension	Systolic ≥ 140 and diastolic <90	

Pre-hypertension

An ideal blood pressure is considered to be below 120/80, with intermediate systolic blood pressure levels of 120–139 mmHg and diastolic pressure of 80–89 mmHg being classed as pre-hypertension. People with pre-hypertension are at increased risk of developing hypertension and should be advised on lifestyle changes and the need for careful follow up. Increased physical activity, weight loss, reduced salt intake and switching to a healthy diet can prevent the development of overt hypertension (see Chapters 10 and 11). At present, there is no evidence to suggest the need to treat pre-hypertension with blood-pressure lowering medications.

White coat (isolated-office) hypertension

It is estimated that up to one-third of people with elevated (≥140/90) clinic blood pressure readings will have normal blood pressure when checked outside the doctor's surgery (office), using either ambulatory or home blood pressure monitors. This is known as white coat or isolated-office hypertension. Blood pressure tends to be higher when recorded outside the home, due to a combination of anxiety and an alert response to an unfamiliar hospital or clinic environment. People who experience white coat hypertension are more likely to have mild hypertension, be female, non-smokers and have no target organ damage. ABPM or HBPM is used to detect white coat hypertension.

5
What causes hypertension?

People with hypertension can be divided into two groups. Most people have hypertension that has no single direct cause, which is called *essential* or *primary* hypertension. In 10 per cent of people, the hypertension is associated with another medical condition that directly causes elevation in blood pressure, for example kidney disease; this is known as *secondary hypertension*. For these people, treating the underlying condition will help lower or normalize blood pressure. Most cases of high blood pressure are due to increases in vascular resistance, as discussed in Chapter 1. The tone and diameter of the arteries and capillaries of the circulatory system are under complex control by hormones (such as angiotensin II and adrenaline), proteins (nitric oxide, endothelin) and nerve inputs (sympathetic and parasympathetic). Any factor that increases vascular resistance can cause hypertension.

Primary (essential) hypertension

High blood pressure in 90 per cent of patients is primary hypertension, which is also known as idiopathic or essential hypertension. This is caused by a combination of multiple genetic and environmental factors and means that there is no single specific cause for high blood pressure that can be reversed, and general blood-pressure lowering treatments are required.

Secondary hypertension

A small proportion (10 per cent) of people with hypertension have a specific underlying (secondary) cause of their high blood pressure. This percentage has not changed over the years, despite improvements in screening for secondary causes of hypertension. Because so many people are affected by hypertension, this small proportion of people affected by secondary causes for hypertension

Table 6 Common secondary causes of hypertension

Secondary cause	Proportion of hypertension patients (%)
Obstructive sleep apnoea	5–15
Chronic kidney disease	1.5–8.0
Primary hyperaldosteronism	1.5–10
Renal artery stenosis	1.0–8.0
Thyroid disease	1–2
Cushing's syndrome	0.5
Phaeochromocytoma	<0.5
Acromegaly	<0.5
Coarctation of the aorta	<1.0

actually account for millions of hypertension patients worldwide; all patients with hypertension should undergo simple screening tests to look for secondary causes (Table 6). The screening involves taking the patient's clinical history, doing a physical examination and performing blood tests, with the possibility of carrying out more detailed investigations if possible secondary causes are identified. It is important not to miss treatable causes of hypertension as appropriate treatment can normalize blood pressure, and prevent the need for long-term drug therapy.

Drug-related hypertension

Several medications can lead to hypertension or make blood pressure treatment ineffective. When your doctor is taking a medical history, he or she should check whether you are taking any of the medications listed below.

- The most common drugs responsible for hypertension are non-steroidal anti-inflammatory drugs (NSAIDs) such as indomethacin and diclofenac. These drugs cause salt and water retention, which increases blood pressure.
- Glucocorticoids (anti-inflammatory steroids) such as prednisolone and dexamethasone also cause salt and water retention.
- Diet pills (phenylpropanolamine and sibutramine) can cause hypertension and doctors no longer prescribe some of these.
- Stimulants (amphetamines and cocaine) cause transient increases

in blood pressure via activation of the sympathetic nervous system.

- Nasal decongestants (containing phenylephrine hydrochloride) are sold over the counter. It is important to mention to your pharmacist that you have high blood pressure as these drugs may not be suitable for you.
- The combined oral contraceptive pill (oestrogen and progestin) induces hypertension in approximately 5 per cent of women. This increase in blood pressure is usually small, although some people may experience severe hypertension. Women taking contraceptive pills undergo regular checks, including blood pressure measurements.
- Antidepressant agents (venlafaxine and monoamine oxidase inhibitors) increase blood pressure in a dose-dependent manner by stimulating the sympathetic nervous system. Reviews for people on these medications should include blood pressure checks as well as discussing their depression.
- The immunosuppressive agent cyclosporin increases blood pressure by activation of the sympathetic nervous system and constriction of blood vessels. Cyclosporin can be prescribed by hospital specialists for several reasons, including to organ transplant patients to prevent rejection of the transplant.
- New targeted anticancer drugs (Avastin and sunitinib) can also cause significant hypertension. These anticancer drugs are developed from synthetic antibodies and target proteins involved in the replication of tumours. Avastin inhibits the vascular epidermal growth factor and sunitinib inhibits tyrosine kinase. These agents are used for certain types of breast, bowel and kidney cancer. Patients treated with Avastin have a five-fold higher incidence of severe hypertension, so people who have been prescribed Avastin should be closely monitored. Once Avastin is no longer taken, people often find that their blood pressure returns to baseline levels.

Obstructive sleep apnoea

Obstructive sleep apnoea is the most common secondary cause of hypertension in adults, accounting for up to 15 per cent of all cases. It is caused by intermittent obstruction to normal breathing during sleep due to collapse of the muscles and soft tissues in the throat. Typically, people with obstructive sleep apnoea complain of exaggerated daytime sleepiness, snoring, morning headaches and poor concentration. Those affected are often male and overweight, tend to have large necks, and may have narrow upper airways. Diagnosis is confirmed by performing overnight monitoring of respiration and blood oxygen levels (polysymnography). Treatment of obstructive sleep apnoea consists of weight loss, avoiding alcohol and sedatives at night and using continuous positive airway pressure (CPAP) facemasks during sleep.

Chronic kidney disease

Chronic kidney disease is the most common cause of hypertension in children. It is the second most common cause in adults. How healthy your kidneys are is important, and, if you have kidney disease, this can cause high blood pressure. This is a double-edged sword as high blood pressure can damage your kidneys. Kidney disease can have mild signs, or none. Although, in more severe cases, symptoms include changes in your body, such as changes to your urine; swelling of your legs, hands or face; tiredness; thirst; and itchy skin. These symptoms mean that at least it is easy to diagnose severe kidney disease so that it can be treated along with the high blood pressure.

The kidneys play an important role in the regulation of blood pressure through salt and water secretion, and also produce several hormones that exert a powerful effect on blood pressure. The hormone renin activates the sympathetic nervous system, as do nerves from the kidneys. Any causes of kidney damage, such as chronic infection, inflammation, scarring, congenital cysts or obstruction, can lead to hypertension. Everyone with hypertension should have a urine test to look for excreted blood, protein and white cells. Creatinine, a waste product, is excreted via the kidneys and is often measured to assess how well the kidneys are working. People with kidney disease often have increased levels of creatinine in their blood.

If you have a suspected kidney problem, other tests that are done might include an ultrasound scan of the renal tract to exclude the possibility of a blockage or obstruction. If a serious problem with your kidneys is suspected, you will need specialist assessment and care from a kidney specialist. The good news is that treating the underlying kidney condition can improve blood pressure control.

Renal artery stenosis

Renal artery stenosis is a condition when one or both of the kidney arteries are narrowed, which can lead to hypertension. In young adults, particularly women, renal artery stenosis can be due to a rare condition called fibromuscular dysplasia, which results in both narrowing and dilatation of medium-sized arteries. The cause is unknown and is thought to be due to a combination of genetic and hormonal factors. The most common cause of renal artery stenosis in older adults is the build up of cholesterol in the arterial wall. This is known as atherosclerosis, or hardening of the arteries, and is the same process that causes heart attacks and strokes. A typical patient with renal artery stenosis may have multiple risk factors for atherosclerosis (including diabetes, hypertension, high cholesterol and being a smoker). Results from blood tests show reduced kidney function and a renal ultrasound will often indicate that there is a smaller kidney on one side. Ultrasound can also identify reduced flow in the renal arteries, although most people require a computerised tomography (CT) scan using X-rays of the renal arteries to confirm the diagnosis.

Some people may be suitable for catheter treatments, which use balloons to dilate the narrowing in the renal arteries. In general, all patients will need to take blood pressure medication. If you have renal artery stenosis, a kidney specialist should manage your treatment; ACE inhibitor drugs, which can cause deterioration in kidney function, should be used with care.

Conn's syndrome

This condition occurs because the body produces too much aldosterone, which is a hormone that controls sodium and potassium levels in the blood. Aldosterone is produced by the adrenal glands, which are found on the upper parts of both kidneys. Although Conn's syndrome is relatively rare, it is always worth investigating to see if it exists in a person, as it is a potentially curable cause of high blood pressure. Symptoms can include intermittent fatigue, muscle weakness, constipation and difficult to control hypertension. Blood tests may show low potassium levels. Diagnosis of Conn's syndrome is made by measuring levels of blood aldosterone and renin, an enzyme secreted by the kidney that breaks down protein and produces a rise in blood pressure (see Chapter 1). Renin levels must be measured before blood pressure treatment is started as some hypertension medications can alter renin levels, which would make interpretation of the results difficult. Surgery may be offered as a treatment, or drugs that inhibit aldosterone action, such as spironolactone, may be prescribed.

Cushing's syndrome

Cushing's syndrome is a rare condition that affects 0.1 per cent of the general population; it is caused by high levels of the hormone cortisol in the body. Common symptoms include weight gain, thinning of the skin and bruising, new stretch marks (stria), fat deposition around the face, which becomes more rounded (moon face) and flushed. Excessive fat around the upper back can lead to a prominent hump, sometimes described as a 'buffalo hump'. People can lose muscle mass in the limbs and complain of weakness. Other symptoms include increased facial hair in women, irregular menstrual periods, acne, and loss of libido. Hypertension is common in people with this condition; hypertension affects around 80 per cent of people with Cushing's syndrome. The most common cause of Cushing's syndrome is drug treatment with corticosteroids such as prednisolone. These drugs are used to reduce inflammation and treat autoimmune conditions in which the body's immune system attacks healthy tissue, such as rheumatoid arthritis and lupus. Cushing's syndrome can also be due to excessive cortisol production caused by pituitary gland tumours; if this is the case, it is known as Cushing's disease or adrenal gland tumours. Treating Cushing's disease may require surgery, if tumours of the adrenal or pituitary glands are involved.

Thyroid abnormalities

The thyroid gland is a very important gland, which is located in the front of the neck. This small butterfly-shaped gland, sometimes known as the powerhouse of the body, controls metabolism by producing a number of different hormones that have key functions in keeping the body healthy. The thyroid produces the hormone thyroxine, which regulates the body's metabolic rate. Both over-production of thyroxine (known as thyrotoxicosis) and under-production (hypothyroidism) can lead to hypertension. A simple blood test can measure thyroid function to easily exclude or diagnose thyroid disease. An underactive thyroid gland often results in symptoms of tiredness, weight gain, constipation, depression and hair loss, because insufficient thyroxine slows the metabolic rate down. However, these symptoms of malaise are common, and not always linked to an underactive thyroid. Other potential causes can include, for example, depression, menopause, anaemia or chronic fatigue syndrome. A blood test will clarify this. An overactive thyroid gland can cause palpitations, sweating, heat intolerance, weight loss, anxiety, diarrhoea, increased appetite and hair loss. This is due to an increase metabolic rate of the body driven by the hormone thyroxine.

Phaeochromocytoma

This is a rare tumour of the adrenal gland, affecting just 0.2 per cent of the general population. Anyone with phaeochromocytoma has high levels of the hormone adrenaline, along with the so-called 'five Ps' – paroxysmal (or intermittent) hypertension, palpitations, perspiration, pallor and a pounding headache. This condition sometimes runs in the family. If your doctor suspects you have it, you will have a urine test to measure levels of catecholamines, which are adrenaline-like hormones that are increased in people with phaeochromocytoma. Phaeochromocytoma is treated with surgery to remove the adrenal glands, after which you will need adrenal hormone supplementation for life, because chemicals released by the adrenal glands are essential to maintain blood pressure and combat stress.

Coarctation of the aorta

This is a rare congenital condition in which there is narrowing (stenosis) of the main artery (aorta), which carries blood from the heart. This condition typically affects young men who have hypertension in their upper limbs and a poor blood supply to their legs. Doctors can diagnose this by feeling the pulse in the groin – a weak or absent pulse is an indication that all is not well with circulation. A CT scan is used to confirm diagnosis, and most people will need surgery or catheter balloon dilatation of the narrowing in the artery.

Acromegaly

Acromegaly is a rare condition caused by excess production of growth hormone from the pituitary gland, resulting in hypertension. Over time too much growth hormone stimulates excess growth of body tissues, leading to enlarged bones, with prominent facial features and large hands. Common clinical signs – that is, what your doctor notes when making a diagnosis – include thickening of the skin and soft tissues, broadening of the nose, prominent bony ridges above the eyes and protrusion of the lower jaw. Those affected may also complain of excessive sweating, acne, joint pain, and symptoms of diabetes (thirst and passing urine more often). People with this condition may also have broad spade-like hands and a large tongue. Acromegaly is also associated with heart failure and an increase in heart size.

Diagnosis is made by testing for high levels of growth hormone. Your doctor may order a glucose tolerance test to check your blood after you have had a sugary drink. Usually, drinking the glucose solution suppresses levels of growth hormone, but in people with acromegaly, the level of growth hormone in the blood will remain high. Your doctor will also measure your insulin-like growth factor (IGF-1) level, which is closely related to insulin; this should rise with the level of growth hormone. Most cases of this uncomfortable condition are due to a benign tumour of the pituitary gland, located below the base of the brain and behind the bridge of the nose. It can be treated by surgical removal of the pituitary gland.

Malignant (accelerated) hypertension

Most people with hypertension have a mild to moderate increase in their blood pressure over many years, with blood pressure levels increasing slowly over time if untreated. As the blood pressure is chronically or consistently elevated, the body adapts to this and many people may remain without symptoms for a long time before complications develop. Malignant hypertension is when people have rapidly increasing blood pressure over a short period. This results in sudden symptoms, such as headache, drowsiness, blurred vision, chest pain, shortness of breath and lethargy. Blood pressure levels are often very high, with systolic readings at more than 200 mmHg, or diastolic more than 120 mmHg. The person may not have any history of hypertension, or, conversely, may not have taken his or her hypertension drugs. Unfortunately, physical examination by your doctor often reveals signs of organ damage

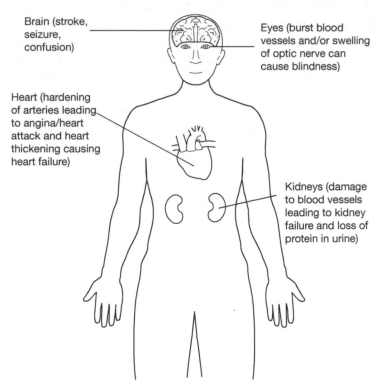

Brain (stroke, seizure, confusion)

Eyes (burst blood vessels and/or swelling of optic nerve can cause blindness)

Heart (hardening of arteries leading to angina/heart attack and heart thickening causing heart failure)

Kidneys (damage to blood vessels leading to kidney failure and loss of protein in urine)

Figure 8 Malignant hypertension symptoms

with haemorrhages and swelling at the back of the eye (retina) and evidence of acute kidney injury (Figure 8). Malignant hypertension is a medical emergency, and if left untreated the prognosis is very poor, with a high mortality rate. There is a serious risk of injury to the small blood vessels in the kidney, eyes and brain (fibrinoid necrosis). As drug treatments take several days to work, urgent hospital admission is needed and people with this condition need to be treated with intravenous drugs to quickly lower their dangerously high blood pressure. Once blood pressure is lowered to safe levels, it is usually possible to achieve long-term satisfactory blood pressure control with drugs for hypertension. Secondary causes for hypertension are more common in people with malignant hypertension. Fortunately with better screening and diagnosis, malignant hypertension is uncommon in western countries.

6

When to treat hypertension

Stage 1 hypertension

You have stage 1 hypertension if your blood pressure readings taken at your GP surgery or hospital clinic are 140–159 mmHg, systolic, or 90–99 mmHg, diastolic; this is equivalent to 24-hour ABPM or home blood pressure measurements of 135–149 mmHg, systolic, or 85–95 mmHg, diastolic. If this is the case, you will be offered advice on your lifestyle. This advice will include the need to take regular exercise, reduce salt intake, avoid excessive alcohol and ensure your diet is rich in fruit and vegetables.

In 2011, in the UK, NICE published guidelines on hypertension recommending that a diagnosis of stage 1 hypertension be confirmed by some form of home monitoring; that is, either ABPM or HBPM. These guidelines also recommend starting treatment to lower blood pressure if there are additional risk factors, including:

- evidence of organ damage, such as damage to kidneys or eyes
- diabetes
- established heart disease or stroke
- kidney disease (with a reduced rate of filtration by the kidneys)
- a high risk of cardiovascular disease.

Mild hypertension – to treat or not to treat

Whereas doctors agree that patients with moderate or severe hypertension should always be offered treatment for hypertension, the benefit of treatment in those with mild hypertension has long been a subject for discussion. The European guidelines (published by the European Society of Cardiology) and US guidelines (published by the American Heart Association (AHA) and the American College of Cardiology (ACC)) have a lower threshold for intervention (that is, they favour prescribing drugs sooner rather than later). These guidelines recommend drug treatment for all patients with stage 1 hypertension if their blood pressure remains high despite lifestyle changes. According to the guidelines, even people with low cardiovascular risk and no evidence of organ damage should be treated. Although there is limited evidence for the treatment of stage 1 hypertension from clinical trials, there are some arguments in favour of initiating treatment. For a start, blood pressure tends to rise with time, and delaying treatment increases the risk to patients. In addition, most drugs for hypertension are well tolerated and many have minimal side effects. They are also inexpensive, which is a necessary consideration for doctors these days.

Older people

Doctors agree that people over the age of 80 with stage 1 hypertension should not receive drug therapy unless blood pressure levels are stage 2 or above. This is based on the lack of evidence for treatment of mild hypertension in the elderly and on the risk of side effects. Postural hypotension is a particular side effect in which blood pressure drops significantly on standing, causing dizziness and, often, distress and discomfort, if not danger, to older people who are more prone to fall.

Stage 2 hypertension

You have stage 2 hypertension if your blood pressure readings taken at your GP surgery or hospital clinic are 160–179 mmHg, systolic, or 100–109 mmHg, diastolic; this is equivalent to 24-hour ABPM or home blood pressure measurements of ≥150 mmHg, systolic, or ≥95 mmHg, diastolic. Everyone with stage 2 hypertension needs drug treatment to reduce blood pressure, irrespective of the presence of additional risk factors.

Severe hypertension

In severe hypertension, your blood pressure readings will be very high whether taken at your GP surgery, hospital clinic or at home, with systolic blood pressure of ≥180 mmHg, or diastolic of ≥110 mmHg. For severe hypertension, treatment should be started without the need for prolonged monitoring. In stage 1 or stage 2 hypertension, it is reasonable to delay treatment while organizing home or ABPM blood pressure monitoring. This will help to exclude people with white coat hypertension, who do need treatment.

Assessing total cardiovascular risk

Cardiovascular disease (CVD) is a term that includes the following events:

- heart attacks
- angina
- stroke and mini-strokes (also known as transient ischaemic attacks or TIAs)
- peripheral vascular disease (compromised circulation in blood vessels in the limbs).

Doctors grade the need for hypertension prevention into two categories, depending on whether you do or do not have heart disease:

- primary prevention – to reduce risk in people who are at risk but do not have established CVD;
- secondary prevention – to reduce the risk of further events in those with established CVD.

Several risk assessment tools are available to help doctors make decisions about the clinical use of blood pressure and lipid-lowering medications for primary prevention. These tools should not be used to make decisions about people with established cardiovascular disease (CVD), whose risk is already considered high enough for them to have to take drugs for hypertension and cholesterol lowering medications.

Recent hypertension guidelines do not focus only on blood pressure as the main factor determining the need for primary prevention treatment. These guidelines have a more integrative approach that estimates an individual's total (global) cardiovascular risk. Hypertension is one of many risk factors for heart disease or CVD. Smoking, diabetes, chronic kidney disease, high cholesterol, family history of CVD, high BMI and a sedentary lifestyle are all associated with increased CVD incidence. A patient-centred approach aims to maintain good cardiovascular health using education and treating all risk factors.

There are many assessment tools that help estimate an individual's 10-year risk of developing CVD. High risk is typically defined as having a score of ≥20 per cent, which means that there is a 1 in 5 chance of suffering from CVD over the next 10 years. The more information you have, the better it is for your health. People at high risk, if given the information on their individual cardio-vascular risk scores, are more likely to stick with lifestyle changes and taking the medications prescribed to them. The most commonly used risk assessment tool in the UK is the QRISK2 calculator (<www.qrisk.org>). QRISK2 is a well-established CVD risk score developed from over 50 million primary care patient records in the UK. It has been used in the NHS since 2009. The current version of the risk calculator takes into account variables that determine your CVD risk including age, gender, family history, diabetes, smoking, cholesterol, BMI, systolic blood pressure, kidney function and heart

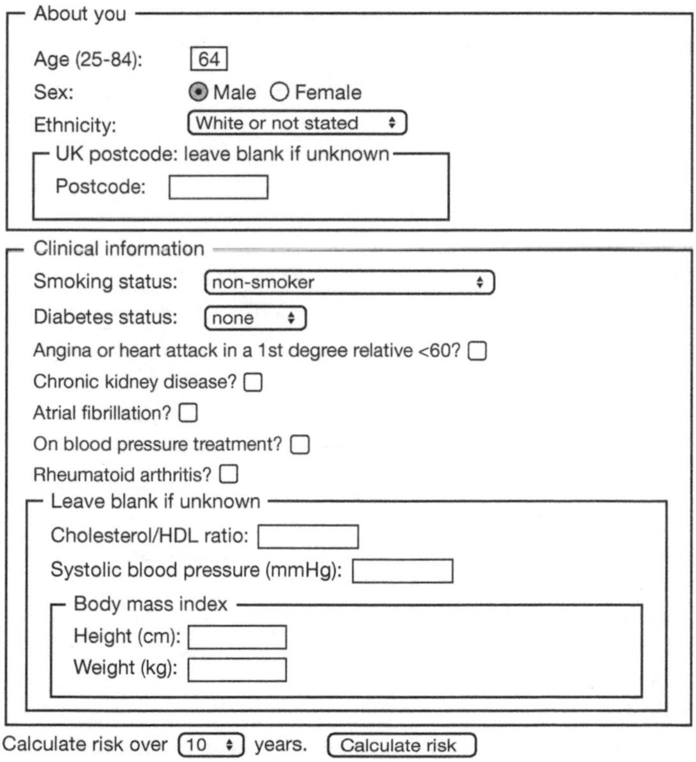

About you

Age (25-84): 64
Sex: ● Male ○ Female
Ethnicity: White or not stated ▼
UK postcode: leave blank if unknown
Postcode:

Clinical information

Smoking status: non-smoker ▼
Diabetes status: none ▼
Angina or heart attack in a 1st degree relative <60? ☐
Chronic kidney disease? ☐
Atrial fibrillation? ☐
On blood pressure treatment? ☐
Rheumatoid arthritis? ☐
Leave blank if unknown
Cholesterol/HDL ratio:
Systolic blood pressure (mmHg):
Body mass index
Height (cm):
Weight (kg):

Calculate risk over 10 ▼ years. [Calculate risk]

Figure 9 QRISK scoring template

rhythm. It can be used for patients taking drugs for hypertension to determine if they need cholesterol lowering-treatment. The calculator includes UK postcode information, which gives a geographical estimate of social deprivation. The QRISK2 calculator is updated every year and is calibrated to the UK population each year (Figure 9 on the previous page).

The Joint British Societies Cardiovascular Risk Prediction (JBS3) Risk Calculator (<www.JBS3risk.com>) was launched in June 2014. This risk tool can also be downloaded as an app onto your phone or tablet. It uses QRISK data to produce an easy-to-understand graph that includes estimates of your 'heart age' and risk of a heart attack or stroke over the next 10 years.

The European guidelines recommend the use of the Systematic Coronary Risk Evaluation (SCORE) calculator.[6] This model uses age, gender, smoking habits, total cholesterol and systolic blood pressure to estimate your risk of fatal CVD disease over the next 10 years (<www.heartscore.org>). The SCORE risk assessment does not take into account level of kidney function, family history or BMI. In the SCORE risk assessment, high risk is defined as a more

Table 7 Diagram of SCORE risk

Number of risk factors plus diseases	Blood pressure			
	High normal	Stage 1 HT	Stage 2 HT	Stage 3 HT
None	–	low risk	moderate risk	high risk
1–2	low risk	moderate risk	moderate to high risk	high risk
≥3	low to moderate risk	moderate to high risk	high risk	high risk
OD, CKD stage 3 or diabetes	moderate to high risk	high risk	high risk	very high risk
Symptomatic CVD, CKD stage ≥4 or diabetes with OD/ risk factors	very high risk	very high risk	very high risk	very high risk

Key CKD, chronic kidney disease; CVD, cardiovascular disease; HT, hypertension; OD, organ damage.

than 5 per cent risk of dying from CVD over the following 10 years. This threshold is different to the QRISK score, which predicts the chances of both fatal and non-fatal CVD, and therefore uses a higher threshold for treatment.

Table 7 shows a simplified version of the SCORE results used to quickly estimate fatal CVD risk (very high, more than 10 per cent; high, 5–10 per cent; moderate, 1–5 per cent; and low risk, less than 1 per cent). Patients with evidence of organ damage, severe kidney failure, symptomatic CVD or diabetes have a very high risk of heart attack or stroke, irrespective of blood pressure. For other patients, the risk increases incrementally as blood pressure rises and/or the number of risk factors increases.

To complicate matters the AHA uses a different CVD risk calculator that also includes race and gender to determine the 10-year risk of first heart attack or stroke (atherosclerotic cardiovascular disease event). The 2013 ACC/AHA Blood Cholesterol guidelines have sparked considerable debate as they recommend a low threshold to initiate lipid-lowering treatments in patients with an estimated 10-year CVD event rate of more than 7.5 per cent.[7] The QRISK, SCORE and AHA risk calculators use different algorithms and have been produced for different populations. They are also useful in determining the need for cholesterol-lowering treatments (such as statins) in hypertensive patients.

The benefits of treatment

Studies have shown that the benefits of treatment are related to the magnitude of blood pressure reduction and not specific to any particular drug. Treatment is beneficial because blood pressure is actually lowered, rather than one or another drug being better or more efficacious. This is because, as far as we know, blood pressure is associated with such a high mortality rate that the benefits of lowering blood pressure remain the most important thing and it doesn't matter which drug is used. This may change in the future as more research is done and new drugs are produced. Using strategies to lower blood pressure within populations could have significant potential health benefits. A reduction in the average population systolic blood pressure by 12–13 mmHg could reduce the incidence of stroke by 37 per cent, coronary heart disease by 21 per cent, death from cardiovascular disease by 25 per cent and all-cause mortality by 13 per cent (Table 8).

Table 8 Benefits of reducing blood pressure in the population

Outcome	Average reduction per 12–13 mmHg decrease in systolic blood pressure (%)*
Stroke	37
Coronary heart disease	21
Deaths from cardiovascular disease	25
Deaths from all causes	13

*These percentages represent the predicted average reduction in disease events in the population achieved by reducing systolic blood pressure by 12–13 mmHg.

7

Drug treatment for hypertension

The development of safe and effective drugs to lower blood pressure has been one of the major breakthroughs in modern medicine. Despite being able to measure blood pressure and monitor its devastating complications since the early 1900s, the options for treatment before the 1960s were limited. One of the most famous patients to suffer from hypertension was President Franklin D. Roosevelt, who died, aged 63, of a brain haemorrhage in April 1945. Hypertension used to be treated with a low-salt diet. Dr Walter Kempner's rice diet programme began in 1939 and consisted solely of white rice, fruit, juice and sugar. Even for those who tolerated this tasteless and monotonous diet, the limited reduction in blood pressure achieved was probably due to weight loss. The only alternative to low-salt diets was bilateral surgical lumbar sympathectomy. This is a major surgical operation that involves cutting the sympathetic nerves from the lower spine to the kidneys and the arteries in the lower limbs. Although blood pressure is significantly reduced, the procedure is poorly tolerated due to severe, disabling drops in blood pressure on standing.

Early medication for lowering blood pressure involved drugs that acted on regions of the brain to cause relaxation of blood vessels (vasodilatation). These 'centrally acting' drugs for hypertension, such as methyldopa, had significant side effects, including constipation, dry mouth, blurred vision and impotence. The first medications to lower blood pressure effectively, without significant adverse side effects, were the thiazide diuretics, which were discovered in 1957. Their discovery was a chance finding by scientists, who noted that patients treated with the antibiotic sulphonamide experienced increased excretion of urine (diuresis). A research chemist, Karl Beyer, through a process of trial and error, modified the formula of sulphonamide to develop chlorothiazide, which is a safe and effective diuretic.

The importance of treatment

No matter how well you feel, it is important for your long-term health that your high blood pressure is treated. Indeed, the most positive aspect of hypertension is that it is a treatable condition with effective medication that is able to prevent unpleasant and life-threatening complications. Clinical trials have convincingly shown that high blood pressure treatments significantly reduce the risk of stroke, heart attack and death compared to dummy (placebo) treatments. The greatest benefit is in stroke prevention. After only one year of treatment for hypertension, blood pressure could be reduced by either 10 mmHg in systolic pressure or 5 mmHg in diastolic pressure with an average 32 per cent reduction in stroke and 20 per cent reduction in coronary heart disease. These results are backed up by the results of long-term trials, and show that the potential effects of blood pressure reduction can rapidly be achieved in just one year.[8]

One of the early trials that looked at the benefits of drug treatment for hypertension was the *US Veterans Administration Cooperative Study on Antihypertensive Agents* published in 1974.[9] This study showed that treating 190 patients with high blood pressure over an average of 3.3 years resulted in a reduction in the number of strokes from 20 to 4. This equated to an 80 per cent absolute reduction in stroke. The authors of the study concluded that 'these results leave little doubt that effective long-term control of hypertension markedly reduces the incidence of stroke in hypertensive patients, particularly with respect to hemorrhagic stroke'.

Patients with very high blood pressure and a history of cardiovascular disease will benefit the most from treatment. It is estimated that treating nine patients for 10 years, with stage 2 hypertension and heart disease, will prevent one death; in comparison, to prevent one death on average, you need to treat 81 patients who have stage 1 hypertension and no cardiovascular disease. In recent years, clinical trials no longer test the effects of treating with blood-pressure lowering drugs against not providing drug treatment and have focused on assessing which of the available drugs works best.

ACE inhibitors

ACE inhibitors were introduced in the early 1980s and are one of the most common drugs used to lower blood pressure. They work by blocking an important enzyme involved in the production of angiotensin II in the kidneys and lungs. Angiotensin II is a powerful hormone that increases blood pressure by causing constriction of the arteries, and increased salt and water retention. ACE inhibitors are also used to protect the kidneys of diabetic patients with kidney disease and treat patients with heart failure. The most common side effect of ACE inhibitors is a dry cough. ACE inhibitors can also cause high potassium levels in those with chronic kidney disease. They can even cause an acute deterioration in kidney function in people with pre-existing narrowed arteries to the kidneys. Blood tests are recommended to monitor potassium levels and kidney function after starting treatment with ACE inhibitors and, if potassium levels rise or kidney function deteriorates after beginning treatment, then treatment should be stopped. Women planning to get pregnant should not take ACE inhibitors, as they can cause foetal abnormalities. Common ACE inhibitors used for lowering blood pressure include ramipril, lisinopril, perindopril and enalapril.

Angiotensin receptor blockers

In the mid-1990s, angiotensin receptor blockers (ARBs) were approved for treating hypertension. This class of medications blocks the receptor that angiotensin II needs to cause salt and water retention and constrict blood vessels. These agents do not cause cough and are better tolerated than ACE inhibitors. They can also be used in diabetic patients with kidney disease and are also used to treat heart failure. ARBs can cause potassium retention and worsening of kidney function in a similar manner to ACE inhibitors, so, again, blood tests to monitor kidney function are required. Common ARBs used to lower blood pressure are losartan, irbesartan, valsartan, candesartan, telmisartan and eprosartan. Each drug has a common generic name and a brand name, which depends upon its manufacturer.

Direct renin inhibitors

The only direct renin inhibitor approved for treating hypertension is aliskiren, which was introduced in 2007. This drug inhibits renin activity, which is an enzyme that controls angiotensin II production. ACE inhibitors, ARBs and aliskiren all work to block the action of angiotensin II. They should not be used together, as any additional benefit is outweighed by the risk of worsening kidney function. In clinical practice, most hypertensive patients will be on either an ACE inhibitor or an ARB; aliskiren has a limited use.

Calcium-channel blockers

Calcium-channel blockers (CCBs) are agents that block the movement of calcium into muscle cells in the heart and into the cells of blood vessels. Calcium plays an important role in controlling muscle tone in blood vessels and heart electrical activity. By slowing calcium movement into cells, CCBs reduce heart rate and cause vasodilatation (opening up blood vessels). Both these actions lead to a reduction in blood pressure. There are two classes of CCBs: dihydropyridine (DHP) and non-DHP CCBs.

- DHP CCBs act mainly on blood vessels and have little effect on the heart. These agents include nifedipine, amlodipine, felodipine and lercanidipine. The main side effect of this group of medicines is ankle swelling, which occurs because of leakage of fluid from cells into the surrounding tissues and is not due to heart failure. Dose reduction can sometimes resolve this swelling. Other less common side effects of these drugs include headaches and flushing.
- The non-DHP CCBs act on blood vessels and also affect heart muscle cells. They cause a slowing of the heart rate and a slight reduction in the contraction of the heart. These agents can also be used for treating heart rhythm disorders. Examples include diltiazem and verapamil. These drugs are less likely to cause ankle swelling; their most common side effect is constipation. Care is required to avoid using these agents with other medications that can slow the heart rate down, such as beta blockers.

Thiazide diuretics

Thiazide diuretics were the earliest drugs to lower blood pressure effectively without disabling side effects. Despite being around for over 40 years, thiazides remain one of the cheapest and most commonly used drugs to treat hypertension. Thiazides work by blocking salt absorption in the distal kidney tubules and increasing excretion of urine (diuresis). They have a relatively weak diuretic effect compared to other 'water pills', such as loop diuretics. Furosemide and bumetanide are commonly prescribed loop diuretics. They block salt transfer across part of the glomeruli, known as the 'loops of Henle', which leads to a significant increase in the volume of urine produced. Blood-pressure lowering occurs because of a reduction in total blood volume and relaxation of arteries. Common thiazide diuretics include bendroflumethiazide, chlorthalidone, cyclopenthiazide, indapamide, metolazone, and xipamide. Thiazides can cause an imbalance in blood salt levels, leading to low sodium, magnesium and potassium levels. If this becomes severe, people can experience weakness, confusion and, in rare cases, heart rhythm disorders. Thiazide medications also increase blood uric acid levels that can precipitate a painful form of arthritis called gout. Thiazides raise blood glucose levels and are associated with a slight increase in the risk of diabetes, or worsening of diabetic control. Men may occasionally experience erectile dysfunction when taking thiazides. Periodic monitoring of blood salt and glucose levels is recommended to prevent these complications, although side effects are infrequent at the low doses that are needed to reduce blood pressure.

Potassium-sparing diuretics

The adrenal glands produce aldosterone that acts on the kidneys to increase salt and water retention, while promoting potassium loss. Diuretics such as spironolactone, amiloride and triamterene increase potassium levels by blocking the action of aldosterone. Potassium-sparing diuretics can be used with thiazide or loop diuretics (in combination) to prevent low blood potassium levels. These are usually chosen in people who have been found to have low potassium levels after taking thiazide alone. Spironolactone is also often used as a third or fourth agent in people with difficult to control (resistant) hypertension, as high aldosterone levels are thought to be one factor responsible for resistant hypertension. Due to their potassium-sparing effects, these agents can cause high potassium levels and blood tests to monitor levels are recommended. Spironolactone can also cause breast enlargement and tenderness (known as gynaecomastia), impotence and menstrual irregularities. Eplerenone is a new aldosterone blocker that does not have the hormonal side effects of spironolactone. It is a useful alternative in people with gynaecomastia caused by spironolactone. Both these agents can also be used in people with heart failure to improve symptoms and the long-term prognosis.

Beta blockers

Beta blockers inhibit the action of adrenaline and noradrenaline (the fight or flight stress hormones) on the heart, blood vessels and kidneys. Beta blockers lower blood pressure by slowing the heart rate, reducing the force of heart contractions, opening up the blood vessels and lowering angiotensin II levels. Beta blockers are often used for people with heart conditions. They are used to treat chest tightness caused by narrowed heart arteries (angina) and can protect the hearts of people with heart failure from the deleterious effects of adrenaline and noradrenaline. Due to their effects on heart rate, beta blockers are used to treat fast heart rhythm disorders such as atrial fibrillation. Commonly used beta blockers include atenolol, bisropolol, carvedilol, metoprolol, nadolol and nebivolol.

Side effects of beta blockers include spasm of the airways, especially in poorly controlled asthma patients in whom they are generally avoided, fatigue, reduced exercise capacity, impotence and having cold extremities. Clinical trials have shown that the beta blocker atenolol is not as effective in preventing stroke as the ARB losartan or the CCB amlodipine, when used as first line treatment for hypertension. The LIFE trial (The Losartan Intervention For Endpoint Reduction in Hypertension Study) compared losartan treatment with atenolol-based treatment for hypertension and thickened heart muscle (hypertrophy). The results were published in 2002 and showed that losartan was superior to atenolol as the group of people who were treated with losartan suffered 25 per cent fewer strokes. This group also had fewer people with diabetes, there was a greater reduction in hypertrophy, and patients in this group showed overall better tolerance to the treatment compared with the atenolol group. These days beta blockers are no longer used as first line agents for the treatment of hypertension, unless patients have concomitant heart failure, angina or heart rhythm problems.

Alpha blockers

Alpha blockers inhibit the action of adrenaline and noradrenaline on the smooth muscle tissue in the walls of arteries. They cause relaxation and dilatation of arteries and lowering of blood pressure. Commonly used alpha blockers include doxazosin, terazosin and prazosin. Alpha blockers are also prescribed for men who have difficulty in passing urine due to enlargement of the prostate. By relaxing the smooth muscles around the prostate, alpha blockers relieve constriction on the urethra and ease urine flow. The main side effects of alpha blockers are dry mouth, headache and dizziness on standing due to a drop in blood pressure (orthostatic hypotension). However, using once-daily slow-release preparations, or taking the medication at night, can reduce dizziness.

Centrally acting antihypertensive drugs

These agents work by inhibiting brain signals that increase blood pressure through activation of the sympathetic system. Examples include methyldopa, moxonidine and clonidine. Side effects are common and can include lethargy, sedation, dry mouth and depression. Poor tolerance means that they are not used as first-line antihypertensive drugs. Methyldopa is still used in pregnant women with hypertension where it is known to be safe and effective.

Aspirin use in hypertension

Platelets are cells in the blood stream that help the formation of blood clots to stop wounds bleeding. However, if clots form abnormally in the circulation, for example, at the site of atheroma (cholesterol deposits) in the heart arteries, they can cause heart attacks. Aspirin blocks the action of platelets and is prescribed, as an antiplatelet drug, to hypertensive patients who have had previous heart attacks or who have significant obstruction of the coronary arteries. The action of aspirin to reduce the formation of blood clots helps to reduce the risk of further heart attacks. The main side effect of aspirin is inflammation of the lining of the stomach, which can cause ulceration and bleeding. Consequently, people who have had peptic ulcer disease or gastric problems should avoid taking aspirin, and because of these side effects there has been a move away from using aspirin as primary prevention therapy in those without symptomatic heart disease, even if they are at increased risk.

Statins

Statins significantly reduce the risk of recurrent cardiovascular events in patients who have a history of heart attack or stroke. Statins are routinely prescribed as part of the secondary prevention therapy in symptomatic vascular disease, to reduce the risk of further events. Statins are also recommended as primary prevention treatment in people without symptoms who are at high risk of cardiovascular events.

Choosing which drugs to take for hypertension

A 10 mmHg fall in systolic blood pressure is associated with a 30 per cent reduction in the risk of death due to a heart attack and 40 per cent reduction in risk of death due to stroke. The drugs routinely used against hypertension are roughly equally effective in lowering blood pressure. The average blood pressure reduction that can be achieved using a single drug is around 9.1 mmHg systolic pressure and 5.5 mmHg diastolic. However, there is a large variation in response between people and some people can have falls in their blood pressure of over 20 mmHg systolic, while other people show very little change.

For most people with hypertension, the blood-pressure lowering effect that can be achieved using a single drug will not be enough to adequately control their blood pressure. Additional treatment options consist of increasing the medication dose, switching to a different agent, or trying two or more drugs in combination. Several studies have shown that increasing the medication dosage only results in a small additional decrease in blood pressure, and that the main treatment effect comes from the initial dose. For example, in a study describing the blood-pressure lowering effects of ARBs, the average blood pressure reduction with 25 per cent of maximum dose was 10.3/6.7 mmHg (systolic/diastolic); with 50 per cent of maximum dose, it was 11.7/7.6 mmHg additional blood pressure reduction, and with the 100 per cent dosage increase it was 13.0/8.3 mmHg.[10] For the thiazide diuretic hydrochlorothiazide, doubling the dose from 25 mg to 50 mg per day led to average blood pressure reduction going from 8/3 to 11/5 mmHg.[11] Therefore, for people with uncontrolled blood pressure, it is better to add a second drug against hypertension, rather than doubling the dose. Using a combination of drugs from two different classes of hypertension drugs can result in a five times greater reduction in blood pressure than doubling the dose of one drug. The ValVET Study, published in 2011, showed that the average systolic blood pressure reduction with an ARB was 9 mmHg, while using an ARB/thiazide diuretic combination led to an average systolic blood pressure reduction of 17 mmHg.[12]

Doubling the dosage of one particular drug is likely to increase the risk of side effects, which often means that people stop taking the prescribed drugs. Over 50 per cent of patients experience ankle swelling when the dose of amlodipine is increased from 5 to 10 mg, and metabolic complications are more common with high doses of thiazide diuretics. The synergist effects of two drugs working together often means that combination therapies are able to achieve reductions in blood pressure that are greater than the sum of the expected reduction achievable with each drug on its own. For example, thiazide diuretics increase angiotensin II levels, which means that ACE inhibitors and ARBs are more effective in lowering blood pressure. If it is proving difficult to achieve an adequate lowering of blood pressure at a reasonable dose, substitution of one drug for one in a different class may be considered. Often it is better to use a second drug especially if blood pressure is significantly above target levels, rather than change drugs.

Different patient groups also respond to drug therapy differently. Elderly patients and patients of African or Caribbean origin are more likely to have 'low-renin' hypertension. This means that their blood pressure elevation is not as dependent on angiotensin II levels as other patient groups, and treatment with CCBs or thiazide diuretics is preferable to using ACE inhibitors or ARBs as an initial therapy.

British Hypertensive Society and NICE guidelines 2011

In the UK treatment for hypertension follows the joint British Hypertensive Society (BHS)/NICE guidelines published in 2011.[13] Many of the recommendations are similar to guidelines published in Europe and the USA. The BHS/NICE guidelines have a simple to follow four-step algorithm that describes the initiation and combination of drug therapy.

- Step 1 – start treatment with an ACE inhibitor or ARB for people ≤55 years of age. For patients over 55 or of African/Caribbean origin, start treatment with a CCB.
- Step 2 – if additional treatment is required, combine the ACE inhibitor/ARB with a CCB.
- Step 3 – if blood pressure remains high, then add in a thiazide diuretic to the ACE inhibitor/ARB plus CCB. Chlorthalidone (12.5–25 mg once daily) or indapamide (1.5 mg modified release or 2.5 mg once daily) are preferred.
- Step 4 – if blood pressure is still high, this is resistant hypertension and referral to a hypertension specialist is advised. Options for additional treatment include spironolactone 25 mg, if serum potassium levels are less than 4.5 mmol/L, increasing the dose of diuretic, or adding in an alpha blocker or beta blocker.

The BHS/NICE guidelines do not recommend thiazide diuretics as drugs to be used in Step 3 due to their adverse metabolic side effects, such as increases in blood glucose levels and a risk of gout. They also have a negative impact on blood lipid levels. US and European guidelines recommend the use of thiazide diuretics earlier than the BHS/NICE guidelines do, as clinical trial data has shown that they are effective at reducing blood pressure and preventing cardiovascular complications. They are also inexpensive and generally well tolerated. The previous BHS/NICE guidelines used to include beta blockers in Steps 1 and 2. However, several clinical trials have shown that the commonly prescribed beta blocker atenolol is not as effective as other medication in reducing the risk of stroke, especially in people aged over 60.[14] The combination of a beta blocker plus a thiazide diuretic should not be used in Steps 1 or 2 as both these drugs increase blood glucose and risk of diabetes.

US guidelines

In April 2014 a scientific advisory statement, *An Effective Approach to High Blood Pressure Control*, from the AHA and the ACC was published.[15] This statement indicates that hypertension is a major modifiable risk factor for CVD and stroke and affects 78 million adults in the USA. Only 53 per cent of hypertensive patients achieve adequate blood pressure control and the quality of treatment varies considerably between different patient groups. Consequently, the AHA and the US Department of Health have made hypertension a primary focus of their strategy to prevent heart attacks and strokes. To improve hypertension treatment, the report recommends following an approach that is similar to the BHS/NICE guidelines, but with some interesting differences.

1 Thiazide diuretics are considered as first line drug therapy along with ACE inhibitors, ARBs and CCBs. The choice is left to the doctor.
2 Lifestyle changes are recommended as an option for people with stage 1 hypertension and drug treatment is considered in all patients if blood pressure remains elevated after three months.
3 For patients with stage 2 hypertension (systolic over 160 mmHg or diastolic over 100 mmHg), initial treatment with a two-drug combination is recommended. Options include thiazide plus either ACE inhibitors, ARBs or CCBs. The alternative option is to use ACE inhibitors plus CCBs.

At present we don't know whether starting treatment with a combination therapy results in better outcomes, compared with the more gradual approach used in the UK. However, we know that at least 50 per cent of hypertensive patients will need more than one drug to achieve adequate lowering of their blood pressure. This strategy may improve blood pressure control by using single pill combination therapies (two medications combined in one tablet).

Single pill combination therapies

It can be difficult sometimes to stick to a drug regime, especially when you need to take several drugs. If you need to take statins to lower cholesterol, and tablets for diabetes alongside your blood pressure drugs, you might find it difficult to take all the tablets. To make life easier and improve people's compliance with their therapies, drug companies have been manufacturing single pill fixed-dose combination therapies. The disadvantages of a fixed-dose combination therapy are that it can be difficult to determine which drug is responsible for any side effects you experience. Also, if your blood pressure remains uncontrolled, it can be difficult to change the dosage of one of the drugs, and combination therapies cost more than taking multiple single drugs. Examples of fixed-dose combination therapies are shown in Table 9.

In my practice, I avoid using a combination of a beta blocker and thiazide due to the increased risk of diabetes. However, this combination may be useful in patients with ischaemic heart disease or heart failure, which provides another reason for using beta blockers. In patients who are intolerant to multiple drugs, beta blocker plus thiazide may be the combination that is used, especially if they are already diabetic.

Blood-pressure lowering targets – the lower the better?

The question that we are always asking ourselves is: what level of blood pressure should we aim for when we treat people with hypertension? You may be surprised to learn that lower is not always better. Lower blood pressure is associated with a lower risk of heart disease. This led to speculation that if it were possible to reduce systolic blood pressure to below 130, rather than below 140, then fewer people would go on to get heart disease. However, clinical trials have shown that for most people this is not the case. The current view is that most benefits from blood pressure reduction occur once blood pressure is no longer at a very high level. As blood pressure falls, there is a threshold below which further reductions only have very small improvement in health outcomes. This relationship between blood pressure and cardiovascular disease is described as a J curve.

In addition, very low blood pressure can have side effects, particularly dizziness on standing. The natural physiological response to standing is for the blood pressure to fall due to pooling of blood in the leg veins. Your body adapts to changes in posture by increasing your heart rate and vascular resistance to maintain your blood pressure when you stand up. Taking medication for high blood pressure will counteract this adaptive reflex and patients on blood pressure tablets often complain of dizziness on standing. Elderly patients

Table 9 Fixed-dose combination therapies

Combination of drug classes used	Trade name	Actual drugs used
ACE inhibitor plus diuretic:	Accuretic	Quinapril plus hydrochlorothiazide
	Capozide	Captopril plus hydrochlorothiazide
	Carace 20 Plus	Lisinopril plus hydrochlorothiazide
	Coversyl Arginine Plus	Perindopril plus indapamide
	Innozide	Enalapril plus hydrochlorothiazide
	Zestoretic 10	Lisinopril plus hydrochlorothiazide
ARB plus diuretic:	CoAprovel	Irbesartan plus hydrochlorothiazide
	Co-diovan	Valsartan plus hydrochlorothiazide
	Cozaar-Comp 50/12.5	Losartan plus hydrochlorothiazide
	Micardis Plus	Telmisartan plus hydrochlorothiazide
	Olmetec Plus	Olmesartan plus hydrochlorothiazide
	Triapin	Felodipine plus ramipril
Calcium-channel blocker plus angiotensin II antagonist:	Exforge	Amlodipine plus valsartan
	Sevikar	Amlodipine plus olmesartan
Calcium-channel blocker plus angiotensin II antagonist plus diuretic:	Sevikar HCT	Amlodipine plus hydrochlorothiazide plus olmesartan
Beta blocker plus diuretic:	Co-tenidone	Atenolol plus chlorthalidone
	Tenoret 50	Atenolol plus chlorthalidone
	Tenoretic	Atenolol plus chlorthalidone
	Kalten	Atenolol plus hydrochlorothiazide plus amiloride
	Prestim	Timolol plus bendroflumethiazide
	Viskaldix	Pindolol plus clopamide

Table 10 NICE blood pressure targets for different age groups

Location of blood pressure reading	Age	Target blood pressure
Clinic	<80	<140/90
	≥80	<150/90
Home or ambulatory blood pressure (daytime average)	<80	<135/85
	≥80	<145/85

are frequently admitted to hospital with falls caused by their blood pressure dropping when they stand up (postural hypotension) and these patients may be advised to stop taking their blood pressure tablets. Most guidelines aim for a target systolic blood pressure of less than 140 and a diastolic blood pressure of less than 90 (Table 10). NICE has less stringent blood-pressure lowering targets for the elderly due to the risk of postural hypotension and lack of evidence for the benefits of a low blood pressure.

Follow up after beginning treatment for hypertension

In most people with hypertension, having their blood pressure taken at the GP surgery is usually enough to monitor their response to treatment. Ambulatory or home blood pressure monitoring can be useful if white coat hypertension is suspected, or where blood pressure remains high despite multiple drugs having been prescribed. If you have been newly diagnosed with hypertension and started on drug treatment, it is important that you are reviewed within two to four weeks to check your blood pressure and assess for possible drug side effects. If your blood pressure remains high, then the available options include adding an additional drug or, occasionally, switching to a different class of hypertension drug. As discussed previously, most people with moderate to high blood pressure do need at least two drugs to achieve satisfactory blood pressure reduction. Once your target blood pressure has been reached, you should be reviewed every six months. If your blood pressure remains stable, your GP should still screen for asymptomatic organ damage and calculate your overall cardiovascular risk every two years.

Is it possible to stop taking hypertension drugs?

Most patients with hypertension will need to stay on drug treatment for life. It is recommended that you do not stop taking your blood pressure tablets without medical advice, as blood pressure can rebound to dangerously high levels. In some people who have good blood pressure control, it may be possible to cut back on the number of drugs taken, especially when taking the drugs has been accompanied by healthy lifestyle changes. As discussed previously, weight loss, increased exercise and reducing your salt intake can all lead to significant reductions in your blood pressure. Any reduction in medication should be done gradually, under the supervision of your doctor, and with careful monitoring of your blood pressure.

8

Resistant hypertension and hypertension in specific patient groups

Resistant hypertension

Approximately 10 per cent of people with hypertension have blood pressure that remains above the target of 140/90 despite taking three different hypertension medications at reasonable doses. These people have resistant, or difficult to control, hypertension. Those with normal blood pressure on four different blood pressure medications are also classed as having resistant hypertension. There are two broad causes of resistant hypertension: apparent or pseudo-resistant hypertension and true resistant hypertension. Pseudo-resistant hypertension may have several causes.

- Non-adherence to medication. Some people don't tell their doctor that they are not taking the prescribed medication (non-compliance). This could be because the drugs have side effects, or these people lack the motivation to take the drugs. They might have a poor understanding of the instructions for taking the drugs, or find the cost of the medications prohibitive, or there may be social barriers that prevent them taking the drugs. In some cases, if the doctor suspects that someone is not taking the prescribed drugs, admission to hospital may be suggested for blood pressure monitoring.

- White coat hypertension. Approximately 25 per cent of those with resistant hypertension will have normal blood pressure if home or ambulatory blood pressure monitoring is used. These people are likely to report symptoms of over-treatment, such as dizziness on standing due to postural hypotension. Chronically elevated blood pressure measured in the GP surgery, without signs of organ damage, is another sign of white coat hypertension.

- Inaccurate blood pressure measurements. Falsely elevated blood pressure readings can be caused by using blood pressure cuffs that are too small. The bladder of the blood pressure cuff should fit snugly, wrapping around at least three-quarters of the upper arm circumference and two-thirds of the length.

True resistant hypertension can be caused by:

- taking medication that causes blood pressure to rise or that interferes with the action of hypertension drugs; these include NSAIDs, steroids (e.g. prednisolone, the oestrogen oral contraceptive pill), or some herbal compounds;
- failure to make lifestyle changes, such as tackling obesity or reducing salt/alcohol intake;
- underlying secondary causes of hypertension, such as chronic kidney disease, obstructive sleep apnoea or Conn's syndrome.

If your doctor suspects that you have resistant hypertension, he or she may:

1 screen for pseudo-resistant hypertension by checking that you are taking your medication as prescribed, and by arranging for you to have ABPM to exclude white coat hypertension;
2 check that you are not taking any other medication that might interfere with the effectiveness of your blood pressure medication;
3 look for secondary causes of hypertension, such as obstructive sleep apnoea;
4 discuss appropriate lifestyle changes with you, especially maintaining a low-salt diet and weight loss, if you are overweight;
5 ensure you are on a drug that addresses the problem of fluid overload, which is common if you have chronic kidney disease. Thiazide diuretics are ineffective at causing diuresis when the filtration rate of the kidneys falls below 30 mL per minute. In patients with resistant hypertension and moderate to severe chronic kidney disease, a thiazide diuretic can be switched to a loop diuretic, such as furosemide. These agents are more potent diuretics and can lower blood pressure due to causing salt and water loss;
6 start low dose spironolactone or another aldosterone antagonist if blood potassium is normal, that is, less than 4.5, with a kidney filtration rate more than 40 mL per minute;

7 add in an alpha blocker or a beta blocker to your medications;
8 consider device-based treatments, such as renal sympathetic denervation, as part of a clinical trial, if previous steps are not successful.

Treatment of hypertension in specific patient groups

Diabetics

In the USA and UK diabetes affects approximately 7–9 per cent of the population. In the USA this equates to around 30 million people, with around one in four US citizens over the age of 65 having a diagnosis of diabetes. Hypertension is very common in diabetes, with approximately 75 per cent of people with diabetes over the age of 18 having high blood pressure. People with diabetes are at increased risk of heart disease, particularly angina and heart attacks. Unfortunately, after a heart attack, people with diabetes tend to be more unwell and have a worse prognosis compared with people without diabetes.

Diabetes is a condition in which the body cannot properly access glucose (sugar), the body's main fuel. Glucose, which comes from food after digestion, normally enters the blood and is used by cells for energy. For this process, the body needs a hormone called insulin, which allows glucose to leave the blood and enter the body's cells. In diabetes, the amount of glucose in your blood is too high because your body cannot use it properly. Uncontrolled diabetes – that is, when blood sugar levels are too high – can cause serious damage to the kidneys, eyes, nervous system, heart and blood vessels. There are two types of diabetes.

- Type 2 diabetes is the most common. This form of diabetes is often related to obesity or a strong family history of diabetes, and is caused by resistance to the glucose-lowering hormone insulin. This means your body either can't make enough insulin, or can't use it. Treatment consists of weight loss, if you are over-weight, with a healthy diet, plenty of exercise and medication to improve sensitivity to insulin.
- Type 1 diabetes accounts for around one in ten cases of diabetes. It occurs when the body is unable to produce any insulin. It is often diagnosed in childhood. Treatment is insulin injections, along with a healthy diet and exercise.

If you have diabetes and high blood pressure, your doctor will want to make sure that your blood pressure is well controlled, and will probably aim for a blood pressure below 130/80, although the benefits of this are not always backed up by clinical research. If you have diabetes and a blood pressure that is consistently 140/90, you will probably be started on drugs to treat your hypertension without delay. Your doctor should also advise you on any necessary healthy lifestyle changes.

All blood-pressure lowering treatments will reduce the risk of heart disease. ACE inhibitors and ARBs are often the first medications tried to lower blood pressure in people with diabetes, as they can also protect against diabetic kidney disease.

Chronic kidney disease patients

High blood pressure and kidney disease often go hand in hand, and, if you have kidney disease, it's vital to ensure your blood pressure is under control, as you are at a higher risk of heart disease or stroke. Hypertension is very common in kidney disease and can cause progressive damage to the kidneys. If you have high blood pressure (more than 140/90) and kidney disease, your doctor will prescribe drug treatment for hypertension. He or she will test for protein in the urine (proteinuria), which is an independent risk factor for heart disease (that is, it is a risk factor for heart disease in its own right along with the well-known risk factors of obesity and lack of exercise) and is thought to signal impaired function of the inner lining (endothelium) of blood vessels.

Protein in the blood is also a marker for more rapid decline in kidney function. Fortunately, there are drugs that work on high blood pressure and on kidney function. ARBs and ACE inhibitors are protective for the kidney and help reduce the level of proteinuria and lower blood pressure at the same time. Clinical trials have shown that these drugs do slow the progression of kidney disease in people with proteinuria, especially when high blood pressure is present. If you have proteinuria, you should have a target blood pressure of less than 130/80; in most people with kidney disease, less than 140/90 is satisfactory.

Older people

The benefits of treating high blood pressure do not stop as you get older, which is fortunate, as older people tend to have high rates of hypertension. Even in people over 80 years old, though, treatment of hypertension is associated with an improvement in survival rates. The Hypertension in the Very Elderly Trial reported that treating high blood pressure in people over 80 years of age resulted in a 21 per cent reduction in mortality, due to lower rates of stroke, heart attacks and heart failure, compared with the placebo treatment.

The disadvantages of treating older people is that they often take multiple medications and are more likely to experience side effects from treatment. Therefore, the balance between risk and benefit needs to be carefully assessed, taking into account blood pressure levels and overall health. In relatively healthy older people, who have blood pressures of 150/90, treatment with a thiazide diuretic and/or with an ACE inhibitor has been shown to improve survival. However, the clinical studies that have looked at treating older people have not included people in nursing homes who have dementia; treatment of hypertension in older people should be considered for each individual and take into account that person's long-term prognosis and overall wishes.

Elderly people are at risk of falls and fractures caused by, for example, arthritis, poor balance and sudden drops in blood pressure on standing up (postural hypotension). The drugs used to treat hypertension can themselves cause postural hypotension and people should be warned that if they experience dizziness on standing, this could be due to a fall in blood pressure. If this happens to you:

- get up carefully;
- if you are lying down, sit up before you stand up, and make sure you move slowly;
- space out taking your hypertensive medication throughout the day.

Children and young adults

High blood pressure in children is diagnosed in a different way than for adults and it is not based on a single cut-off reading over 140/90.

At least three high readings on separate occasions are needed to make the diagnosis. Most cases of hypertension in children are related to lifestyle issues, particularly obesity. Secondary causes are more common than in adults, but are still only responsible for a small overall percentage of children with high blood pressure. Chronic kidney disease is one of the most common secondary causes of hypertension in children. High blood pressure in children often leads to hypertension in adulthood and strategies to lower blood pressure may prevent people developing hypertension in later life.

Overweight hypertensive children should be encouraged to increase levels of physical activity and reduce calorie intake. It is estimated that 3 per cent of children between 3 and 18 years of age have hypertension and around 30 per cent of obese adolescents have either blood pressure at the upper normal range or hypertension. Measurement of blood pressure in children is not routine practice and more children may have high blood pressure than is known. Only a few clinical trials have examined treatments for high blood pressure in children and so there are only a few evidence-based recommendations, although clinical experience suggests that persistent hypertension in children should be treated with drugs. Current risk prediction methods are likely to underestimate the lifetime risk for cardiovascular disease in young adults with high blood pressure, and the decision to treat should incorporate the presence of additional risk factors and evidence for target organ damage. Ambulatory or home blood pressure monitoring is useful to exclude white coat hypertension and monitor the results of treatment.

Drug treatment to lower blood pressure is challenging in young adults as managing to take the prescribed medication can be difficult, and it is often the case that these young adults will need to remain on lifelong therapy, which can be difficult for them and their parents to come to terms with. Young female patients need to be advised that many hypertension treatments, including ACE inhibitors, ARBs and thiazide diuretics, should not be taken in case of pregnancy as they can have harmful effects on the foetus.

Hypertension in pregnancy

Around one in 20 women develop high blood pressure during pregnancy, when the cardiovascular system has to work harder to meet the increased metabolic needs of the mother and baby. Heart rate and heart contraction increase, while blood pressure falls, particularly during the first half of pregnancy.

High blood pressure during pregnancy can be dangerous for both mother and baby. High blood pressure can impair the baby's growth in the womb and lead to premature delivery. It also increases the risk of stroke and placental bleeding in the mother, and routine monitoring of blood pressure in pregnancy is a very important component of good antenatal care. Some women already have high blood pressure (chronic hypertension) that is present before pregnancy or is detected during the first half of pregnancy. In these cases, blood pressure remains high after pregnancy and long-term follow up is needed. Women with pre-existing hypertension usually do well with a target blood pressure during pregnancy of less than 150/100. ACE inhibitors and ARBs should ideally be stopped before pregnancy as they increase the risk of congenital abnormalities. Thiazide diuretics can potentially cause foetal abnormalities, and the safest drugs to use are nifedipine (a calcium-channel blocker), labetalol (a beta blocker) and methyldopa.

Gestational hypertension is new hypertension that is diagnosed after 20 weeks of the pregnancy. If you have protein in your urine along with high blood pressure, there is a high risk of pre-eclampsia. Pre-eclampsia is a serious condition that affects around 5 per cent of all pregnancies, usually after 34 weeks. It can cause serious maternal and foetal complications, especially when the blood pressure is very high (that is, more than 160/110). It involves possible damage to the endothelium – the tissue that forms the lining of cells and various organs in the body, such as the blood vessels, lymphatic vessels and heart. Pre-eclampsia can also cause damage to the mother's kidneys and liver. Women with pre-eclampsia may need hospital observation and specialist care. The only cure for pre-eclampsia is to deliver the baby; the timing of delivery is determined by the severity of the condition and the maturity of the baby. If you have high blood pressure and are considering getting pregnant, it's important that you discuss the matter with your doctor first. He or she can then help you to get your blood pressure under control before and during the pregnancy. I would advise that you make determined efforts to avoid pregnancy until your blood pressure is under control. This will involve making sure that you are leading a healthy lifestyle by limiting the salt in your diet, stopping smoking, taking regular exercise, avoiding alcohol and eating a healthy diet. If you are overweight it will also help you if you drop to a more healthy weight for your height. If you take medication to control your blood pressure, it's important that you discuss this with your doctor while planning your pregnancy.

Blood pressure treatment after stroke

High blood pressure is the most important modifiable risk factor for stroke. Around 90 per cent of all strokes are caused by a blood clot blocking a brain artery (ischaemic stroke) and causing permanent brain damage. Stroke can also be caused by small blood vessels in the brain bursting and bleeding, which is called haemorrhagic stroke. After an acute stroke, blood pressure can increase significantly but it usually settles spontaneously in the first seven days. It is not known whether elevated blood pressure is a protective response to the stroke or whether it occurs due to stress caused by brain injury. The current opinion is not to treat high blood pressure soon after a stroke, although this topic is the subject of ongoing clinical trials and debate. In patients who had hypertension before their strokes, oral medication should be started again as soon as the patient can swallow, so long as systolic blood pressure is not below 110. In patients with no prior history of hypertension, it is reasonable to wait seven days. If systolic blood pressure remains above 120/70 mmHg, drug treatment for high blood pressure is advisable to reduce the risk of further stroke; this treatment threshold is lower than the blood pressure threshold for non-stroke patients. Most of the hypertension drugs can be used apart from beta blockers, which are less protective for the brain owing to their limited effect on central (aortic) blood pressure.

If the stroke is caused by a clot from the heart caused by an irregular pulse (atrial fibrillation), the threshold for treatment is a blood pressure of more than 140/90. These patients need to take long-term blood thinners (anticoagulants) once they have recovered from the acute stroke. Statin drug therapy is also recommended after an ischaemic stroke, which is often caused by fatty deposits (atherosclerosis) in the lining of brain arteries.

Statins not only lower blood cholesterol, but also have additional properties including stabilization of plaques in the arterial wall, reduced arterial inflammation and improvement in arterial function.

Blood pressure treatment after heart attack

Heart attacks happen when there is a sudden complete or near complete blockage (occlusion) of the heart artery. This results in lack of blood and nutrients being supplied to part of the heart muscle, which then starts to die. The blockage in the heart artery is made up of fatty plaques in the artery wall (atherosclerosis) and occlusive blood clots. Treatment for a heart attack has three components.

- First, patients need to be given drugs that reduce the clotting ability of the blood to try and open the blocked artery. Medication, such as aspirin and clopidogrel, inhibit platelets from forming clots. Additional blood thinners (anticoagulants), similar to heparin, are also prescribed.
- Second, doctors attempt to limit the amount of heart muscle damage. In patients with a complete occlusion of the heart artery, the electrical tracing of the heart (electrocardiogram or ECG) shows the changes typical of this condition. Patients with 'ST elevation' changes need emergency treatment as soon as possible to open the blocked heart artery. In modern healthcare systems, this involves transfer to a cardiac centre for emergency coronary angioplasty, a minimally invasive procedure where a catheter is placed, via an artery in the wrist or groin, into the heart arteries and equipment such as stents can be delivered to treat the occlusion. The most common type of heart attack is a 'non-ST elevation' heart attack, where there is often a severe narrowing in the heart artery without total occlusion. In this situation, coronary angioplasty can be delayed and performed within 24–72 hrs after admission in stable patients.
- Third, adequate control of blood pressure, and additional risk factors, must be achieved to prevent further heart damage. Medications such as ACE inhibitors or ARBS are often prescribed to limit the progression of atherosclerosis and reduce blood pres-

sure. These drugs are also useful in cases of heart failure when there has been a significant decline in heart pump function. Beta blockers are protective for the heart after a heart attack, especially when blood pressure is elevated or there are signs of heart failure.

All patients with a heart attack are prescribed statins, which have been shown to improve long-term survival and reduce the risk of another heart attack. Target blood pressure after a heart attack should ideally be less than 140/90, with most patients being discharged with ACE inhibitors and beta blockers, irrespective of their blood pressure.

Management of hypertension during surgery

Uncontrolled blood pressure is a major risk factor for acute heart complications and bleeding during surgery, and poorly controlled hypertension is a common medical reason to postpone elective surgery, that is, non-emergency surgery. Before elective surgery, your blood pressure should be below 180/110, and ideally below 140/90. If emergency surgery is necessary, then a patient with a very high blood pressure can be treated with medications given via a drip directly into the veins (intravenous) to bring the blood pressure down to safe levels. Patients taking hypertension medications should not stop treatment before surgery. Normal medications can be taken with a sip of water in the morning after discussion with the surgical team. Treatment can then be resumed after surgery when normal oral intake is allowed. Blood pressure can be elevated post-surgery due to pain, agitation or bladder distension. If blood pressure remains very high (that is, more than 180/110) with no reversible cause then initiation or intensification of hypertensive drug treatment may be required.

When you might need specialist advice

Most people with high blood pressure are well managed by their GPs and do not need to see hospital specialists. Referral to a hypertension specialist (usually a cardiologist) is sometimes needed for the following reasons:

- if you have resistant hypertension; that is, your blood pressure remains elevated despite taking three different hypertension drugs, including a diuretic;

- if you are under 40 and have hypertension, as screening for a secondary cause for high blood pressure is needed;
- if your GP suspects that you have secondary hypertension;
- if there is evidence of target organ damage, such as left ventricular hypertrophy, heart failure or significant kidney disease
- if you are intolerant to several hypertension drugs and have difficulty in achieving your target blood pressure.

Advances in hypertension treatment – renal sympathetic denervation

High blood pressure is usually treated using medication and lifestyle change, and historical surgical treatments for hypertension, which targeted the sympathetic nervous system, have been abandoned due to development of well-tolerated drugs and the high complication rate with surgery. In 2009 the Symplicity HTN-1 study reported the results of a new surgical technique to target the sympathetic nerves. This minimally invasive technique is performed in a procedure similar to a coronary angiogram. With the patient under local anaesthesia, a catheter is inserted from the femoral artery in the groin, and the tip of the catheter can be positioned in the artery to one of the kidneys. This is done under X-ray guidance. By delivering energy to the tip of the catheter, which is slowly rotated to produce a series of lesions, the sympathetic nerves running on the outside of the kidney artery can be permanently damaged. The procedure takes around 1 hour to complete and both kidney arteries are treated in turn. The technique is thought to work because the sympathetic nerves from the kidney are important in controlling blood pressure. By reducing sympathetic flow from the kidneys, blood pressure can be effectively and permanently reduced.

The Symplicity HTN-1 study showed that in patients with drug-resistant hypertension, this technique produced a mean reduction in blood pressure of 23/11 mmHg that lasted at least 12 months. The initial small non-randomised study included only 45 patients. However, the results generated a lot of interest and a second larger randomised study (Symplicity HTN-2), involving 106 patients from 24 centres, confirmed the initial findings. Scepticism was replaced with enthusiasm and the procedure was offered in many centres throughout Europe with thousands of patients undergoing the treatment. A large, multinational medical device company acquired, for several hundred million dollars, the business that had initially developed the renal denervation catheters. Other medical device companies scrambled to produce their own catheters for this treatment and research into renal denervation increased dramatically.

The US Food and Drug Administration requested that a large, well-performed study should be conducted before the treatment could be recommended in the USA. In March 2014, the results of the Symplicity HTN-3 trial were published in the *New England Journal of Medicine*.[16] This large randomised trial with 535 patients included a 'sham control' group, which was not present in previous studies. This meant that although all patients underwent a procedure, the 'sham control' group had images of the kidney arteries taken but no treatment was performed. Importantly, patients did not know if they were in the control or treatment group. Also, ABPM was used to screen patients for true resistant hypertension. The medical community was surprised by the results. There were no significant medical differences in the average blood pressure reduction seen in the sham control and treatment groups. The mean reduction in systolic blood pressure was 12 mmHg for the sham control group and 14 mmHg for the treatment group, meaning that both groups experienced a significant reduction in blood pressure compared to baseline values. Several mechanisms have been postulated to explain these findings. The placebo effect could explain the fall in blood pressure in the control group. The placebo effect is when patients feel better due to the perceived benefits of treatment rather than due to an active drug or therapy. The experience of undergoing a procedure can produce powerful physiological and psychological responses. Another possible explanation is that patients change their behaviour when taking part in a clinical study. They start to take their medications regularly and are more motivated to make positive lifestyle changes.

Not surprisingly, the future for renal denervation has been seriously set back by the results of this latest study. At present the procedure is still being offered in some centres as part of ongoing, carefully conducted research. However, one benefit of renal denervation has been to refocus research on the importance of the sympathetic system in the regulation of blood pressure.

9

Lifestyle issues that affect your blood pressure

Hypertension is the most common risk factor for stroke and the leading global cause of premature death. Fortunately, there are many lifestyle and drug regimes that can help reduce your blood pressure and lower the risk of cardiovascular complications. So, what lifestyle changes can you make? First and foremost comes exercise, with one of its main values in blood pressure control being to aid weight loss, and even small amounts of weight loss have a positive impact on blood pressure.

Exercise

People who take exercise have lower average blood pressure and are less likely to develop high blood pressure than those who are sedentary. Being active and taking regular exercise conditions the heart and cardiovascular system so that oxygen can be transported around the body more efficiently. Indeed, people who are physically active are 20 to 50 per cent less likely than their sedentary counterparts to develop high blood pressure. Exercise is therefore a powerful weapon against the condition, particularly when adopted in conjunction with other measures such as a healthy diet, stress control and medication, if necessary. Whether you are at risk of high blood pressure, or have actually been diagnosed with the condition, you can significantly lessen your risk of the condition developing by following a regular exercise regime. Long-term regular exercise has been shown to reduce the risk of death due to cardiovascular disease. The benefits of exercise include:

- lowering blood pressure;
- preventing the development of diabetes;
- reducing cholesterol levels;
- helping to maintain a healthy weight.

Regular physical activity can lower systolic blood pressure by as much as 5–15 mmHg in people with hypertension. A similar fall in blood pressure has been seen in those with borderline hypertension, where exercise can lower blood pressure well into the normal range.

Both aerobic exercise such as running, cycling or swimming and resistance training using weights are effective in lowering blood pressure. Exercise helps to rebalance our autonomic nervous system, by reducing sympathetic and increasing parasympathetic activity. The net result is a lowering of pressure by decreasing both vascular resistance and force of the heartbeat. The blood pressure response to exercise is dependent upon maintaining a regular exercise programme, and stopping exercise results in a return of blood pressure to pre-exercise levels. The good news is that the beneficial effect of exercise on blood pressure reduction is related more to the intensity of training rather than the frequency. One hour of moderate-intensity exercise split over two sessions seems to be as effective as two hours per week of low-intensity exercise. The traditional teaching is that hypertensive patients should undertake 30 minute of moderate-intensity aerobic exercise (walking, jogging, cycling or swimming) five times per week. It does not take much effort to become more physically active. You can divide 30 minutes into 10-minute sessions spread throughout the day. This can include walking or cycling to work, using the stairs instead of a lift, or taking a brisk walk during lunch.

Similar beneficial effects on blood pressure can be achieved with 75 minutes of vigorous intensity exercise spread throughout the week. Moderate exercise is any exercise where you increase your heart rate to between 50 and 70 per cent of maximum, which means that you should be able to exercise and talk at the same time. With vigorous exercise, the increase in heart rate is 70–85 per cent of your maximum heart rate, and you can only say a few words before stopping for breath while exercising. Your maximum predicted heart rate during such exercise is calculated to be 220 beats per minute minus your age (220 – age, in years). Emerging clinical data suggests that high intensity training (HIT) may be as effective or better than moderate-intensity training for lowering blood pressure. Here are some points to consider before you exercise.

- Choose your type of exercise with care and avoid any activity that may be difficult to keep up, such as expensive gym membership or rowing at a club a long way from home. It may be better to have two or three exercise possibilities to hand, such as gardening, walking and playing tennis, as variety makes exercise more interesting and more likely to be kept up. When considering exercise possibilities, prioritise the ones you think you can easily do and start slowly and gently, especially if you are out of the habit of exercising. It's not wise to throw yourself straight into a more challenging routine. Consult your doctor if in any doubt, particularly if you are overweight or have not exercised for some time.

- If your doctor recommends that you carry out only gentle exercise, remember that after following the guidelines in this book, your blood pressure may drop to a level at which you may safely increase your level of exercise if you wish.

- Studies have shown that people with blood pressure in the normal to high range who perform moderate-intensity cardiovascular exercise for 45 minutes per day, at least three times a week, have a reduction in blood pressure at rest and during moderate exercise. The types of exercise carried out in these studies were brisk walking, jogging, gardening and housework.

How soon does exercise take effect?

Most studies into the effects of exercise on high blood pressure have shown that the body responds quickly – there can be a notable drop in blood pressure in the very first week, with further falls occurring a few weeks later. However, if you stop exercising, blood pressure rapidly soars again and returns to its pre-exercise status. This means that exercise must be taken regularly for continued benefits, and is another reason why it's important to choose something that you can adopt easily and maintain without too much effort.

Can older people exercise?

Yes, certainly, though you should check with your doctor first, especially if you have not taken exercise for some time. In studies, older patients with high blood pressure carried out both aerobic exercise and weight training for three hours per week, with no adverse effects on diastolic blood pressure or heart function at the end of the programme. Indeed, for most participants their blood pressure decreased. Other positive effects were an approximate 20 per cent reduction in abdominal fat, together with an average weight loss of 2.2 kg (4 lb).

Diet and weight

What a person eats and drinks has an effect on overall health as well as on heart and blood pressure. For blood pressure, the most important component here is body weight. A junk food diet, with high levels of sugar and salt, chemical additives, and refined carbohydrates (such as cakes, pastries, biscuits, sweets, sweetened fruit juices) and so on, is highly likely to push weight up to unhealthy levels, making high blood pressure (and other health issues) more likely. A balanced whole food diet, on the other hand, with plenty of fresh fruit and vegetables, is far more effective at promoting and maintaining a healthy weight.

Obesity

The rising prevalence of obesity in both adults and children has been described as a global pandemic. In the USA, approximately one in three adults is obese and one in five adults in western Europe is obese. A combination of high-calorie fast food diets, limited consumption of natural (non-processed) foods, sedentary routines and lack of exercise are all contributing to increasing obesity. Obesity is an important risk factor for elevated blood pressure and increases the risk of all causes of mortality. It is also associated with higher rates of diabetes and elevated blood cholesterol levels. Being overweight more than doubles a person's chances of developing high blood pressure. About 70 per cent of overweight adults already have high blood pressure and a blood pressure reading generally corresponds with the degree of obesity. The rise in blood pressure with obesity is due to the increased force of heart contraction and vascular resistance needed for the body to generate the pressure required to push blood around an increased body size. BMI is the standard method for assessing obesity because it takes into accounts both weight and height (Table 11).

BMI, however, is not always a reliable guide to obesity, as it may overestimate body fat in very muscular people or in people who

Table 11 Body size definitions using BMI

Body size	BMI (kg/m²)
Normal	18.5–24.9
Overweight	25–29.9
Obese	30 or above
Morbid obesity	40 or above

have a lot of swelling due to fluid (oedema). Conversely, BMI may underestimate body fat in people with significant muscle wasting or older people. BMI also estimates total body fat with no regard to how the fat is distributed.

Measuring fat around the waistline is a useful addition to the BMI, with guidelines suggesting a target waist circumference of less than 104 cm (40 inches) for men and 88 cm (35 inches) for women; 90 cm (35.5 inches) for Asian men and 80 cm (31.5 inches) for Asian women. Fat around the waist (known as central obesity) is especially detrimental to health, and is associated with a high risk of cardiovascular disease. As well as the extra weight you can see, invisible extra fat inside the body affects your health. Central obesity is linked to increased fat inside your middle, which accumulates around the vital organs in the abdomen and secretes several hormones that induce an adverse metabolic profile. This is linked to the development of hypertension, type 2 diabetes and high cholesterol levels.

On the positive side, losing weight does have an impact on blood pressure. In overweight people with hypertension, a 1 kg reduction in weight is associated with an average reduction of 1–1.5 mmHg in systolic blood pressure. In my own clinical practice, I have noticed an increase in referrals of young patients with hypertension. A significant number of these patients are obese with no other cause for hypertension, and it is likely that weight loss would normalize their blood pressure. As even a small amount of weight loss can bring down your blood pressure, it really is well worth making every effort to lose some weight and pre-empt the need for lifelong medication. A reasonable target is for 5–10 per cent of weight loss over a six-month period. This can be achieved by creating an energy deficit through a combination of reduced calorie intake and exercise. For the average adult, a calorie intake of 1,500 kilocalories per day will result in an energy deficit of 500 kilocalories. If sustained over one week, this should result in loss of one pound of body weight.

- Changing to healthy eating will result in weight loss. Rather than feeling you have to go hungry, aim to think about eating healthy foods for the rest of your life.
- Do not consider crash dieting or trying to follow a 'fad' diet such as the cabbage soup diet – they are impossible to maintain on a lifelong basis and can be dangerous, too. The 5/2 diet has become popular in recent years (fasting for two days of the week and eating for the other five). Again, approach this with caution and consult your doctor before making any drastic changes in your diet.
- If you have adopted a healthy eating diet but are not losing weight, aim to have smaller helpings of calorie-dense foods such as meat and cheese and avoid returning for seconds. You may also need to increase your physical activity.
- Write down what you eat and when you eat it, too. Snacking without really being aware of it accounts for a great deal of 'inexplicable' weight gain, especially if you snack on high-calorie foods such as crisps and chocolate instead of fresh fruits. *My Fitness Pal*, www.myfitnesspal.com, has a free calorie counter and is a useful tool for keeping track of your food intake in this way.

Lifestyle changes are difficult to implement without support. Regular individual or group meetings with dieticians or support workers as part of a comprehensive lifestyle programme can significantly improve motivation and results, so if your own measures are not successful, do ask your doctor for further help and advice.

The DASH diet

A variety of dietary approaches can lead to weight reduction as long as your total energy intake is reduced. Do bear in mind that your diet can also help to lower blood pressure. The Dietary Approaches to Stop Hypertension (DASH) diet is recommended by the AHA to prevent and control hypertension. The DASH diet emphasizes the need to eat vegetables, fruit and low-fat dairy foods along with moderate amounts of whole grains, fish, poultry and nuts. It is low in red meat, sugary drinks, sweets and fat. This contrasts with the typical American diet where 63 per cent of daily calorie intake comes from processed foods with added sugar, fat, oils and refined grains. Plant foods (fruit and vegetables) only make up 12 per cent of daily calorie intake, with 25 per cent coming from animal food sources (meat, fish, eggs and dairy).

A typical daily menu on the DASH diet would include 2 cup-sized portions of fruit, 2 cup-sized portions of vegetables, 6 oz of grains (preferably whole grains), 2 small portions of lean meat or fish and 2 cup-sized portions of low-fat dairy food with limited fat and sugar intake. This should be supplemented with 4–5 servings of nuts, seeds and legumes per week. Over a 3-month period a combination of a low-sodium diet and the DASH diet has been shown to reduce blood pressure by an average of 11/6 mmHg in patients with hypertension (Figure 10).

Below are other ways in which you can eat more healthily.

- Eat more fruit and vegetables. Fruit and vegetables are rich in vitamins, minerals, fibre and enzymes, and can help to lower blood pressure.
- Fruit such as bananas, prunes, cantaloupe and honeydew melon and dried peaches and apricots are high in potassium.
- Eating onions, celery and garlic on a daily basis has been shown to reduce systolic blood pressure in people with high blood pressure.

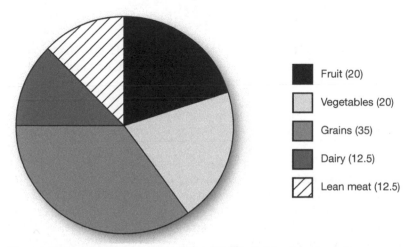

Figure 10 Daily components of the DASH diet (percentages)

- Try to eat food as fresh and as raw as possible. When you have to cook your vegetables, use unsalted water and simmer lightly, steam or stir-fry.
- Don't soak prepared fruit or vegetables as the vitamins and minerals can dissolve away.
- Don't buy vegetables that come with sauces. These sauces are likely to contain a lot of added salt, sugar or fats.
- Frozen, dried and tinned vegetables are acceptable substitutes to fresh vegetables, provided they don't contain added salt and sugar.

Whole grains

Eat wholegrain and wholemeal flours to help you to achieve your optimum weight. For each daily serving of wholegrain, your chance of developing high blood pressure is likely to fall by about 4 per cent. People who consume four servings a day are as much as 23 per cent less likely to develop the condition. When you also take other steps to lower your blood pressure, the estimated drop in your risk of getting high blood pressure is even greater.

Aim to consume a variety of grains, with the exception of wheat, including oats, rye, barley (generally available as pearl barley), corn, buckwheat, brown rice and mixed grains. Brown rice, millet, buckwheat and maize or corn are all gluten-free and invaluable to people with a gluten allergy or sensitivity.

Here are some further tips for eating wholegrain:

- a morning bowl of porridge is an excellent start to the day;
- use brown rice instead of white, and wholewheat pasta instead of refined white pasta;
- use wholegrains such as barley in soups and stews;
- use bulgur wheat in casseroles and stir-fries;
- make a pilaf with wholegrains such as wild rice, brown rice and barley;
- substitute half the refined white flour in pancakes, buns and other flour-based recipes for wholewheat or oat flour;
- use rolled oats or crushed unsweetened wholegrain cereal to coat chicken, fish, veal cutlets and so on;
- use wholegrain flour or oatmeal when baking, for example, scones, cakes and crumbles.

- Legumes (peas and beans) are inexpensive, versatile and contain high amounts of protein, which is vital to the body for growth and maintenance. They can be used in salads, curries and as meat substitutes in dishes such as lasagne and shepherd's pie.
- Sunflower, sesame, hemp, flax and pumpkin seeds can be eaten as snacks, sprinkled on to salads and cereals, or used in baking. For more flavour they can be lightly roasted and coated with organic soy sauce. Cracked linseed and pumpkin seeds are also highly nutritious and are useful for treating constipation. They can be used in baking and sprinkled on to breakfast cereals, over salads, soups and porridge oats.
- Nuts contain vital nutrients; almonds, cashews, walnuts, Brazil nuts and pecans perhaps offer the greatest array of nutrients. Eat a wide assortment of nuts as snacks, with cereal and use them in baking (unless you are allergic to nuts, of course).

How much is a portion of fruit and vegetables?

One portion of fruit or vegetables weighs about 80 grams (just under 3 oz) and is roughly the size of your fist. For example, a portion might be:

- one medium-sized fruit (banana, apple, pear, orange)
- one slice of a large fruit (melon, pineapple, mango)
- two smaller fruits (plums, satsumas, apricots, peaches)
- a dessert bowl full of salad
- three heaped tablespoonfuls of vegetables
- three heaped tablespoons of pulses (chickpeas, lentils, beans)
- two or three tablespoons of grapes or berries
- one tablespoon of dried fruit
- one glass (150 ml or 5 fl oz) of unsweetened fruit or vegetable juice. (If you drink two or more glasses of juice, it still only counts as one portion.)

Salt restriction

The typical western diet contains 9–12 grams of salt, which is more than twice the recommended daily allowance. It is estimated that the body requires less than 1 gram of salt intake a day to maintain healthy function. There is good evidence to suggest that excessive salt intake can lead to the development of high blood pressure.

Population studies have shown that high salt intake is associated with an increased prevalence of hypertension. Clinical trials have also shown that reducing salt intake from 8 to 4 grams a day will on average reduce systolic blood pressure by 7 mmHg, and diastolic blood pressure by 3.5 mmHg. Salt works on the kidneys to increase fluid retention and also vascular resistance, thereby increasing blood pressure. High salt intake not only adversely affects the heart, blood vessels and kidneys, but also is linked to kidney stones, asthma, osteoporosis and stomach cancer. A reduction in dietary salt intake is therefore an important means of treating and preventing hypertension and other conditions.

The guidelines on salt intake are confusing because some countries look at sodium levels instead. The chemical name for salt is sodium chloride (chemical formula $NaCl$). To convert sodium into salt, you need to multiply the amount of sodium by 2.5. Therefore:

- 1 gram salt = 400 milligrams (mg) sodium (a good pinch of salt)
- 2.5 gram salt = 1,000 mg sodium (1/2 teaspoon)
- 5 gram salt = 2,000 mg sodium (one teaspoon)
- 6 gram salt = 2,400 mg sodium.

The effect of salt reduction on blood pressure is more pronounced in patients with kidney disease, the elderly, diabetics and patients of African origin. Reduced salt intake also increases the blood-pressure lowering effects of medications that block the RAAS system, such as ACE inhibitors and ARBs.

The current recommended salt intake is up to 6 grams per day. The UK's National Institute for Health and Care Excellence aims to reduce salt intake further to less than 4.8 grams per day by 2015 and less than 2.4 grams per day by 2025, with lower targets in children. The AHA has lowered its recommended daily sodium intake from 2,300 mg (5.8 gram salt) to no more than 1,500 mg (3.8 gram salt). Lowering salt consumption is one of the AHA's major priorities in reducing deaths from cardiovascular disease and stroke. Salt restriction is a very important component of a healthy diet. However, cutting back on salt is not easy, as approximately 80 per cent of dietary salt is contained in processed supermarket foods or restaurant meals. The food categories that contribute most to salt intake – the Salty Six – are: breads and rolls, cured meats and cold cuts, pizza, poultry, canned soups, and burgers and sandwiches (Table 12).

Table 12 The six most common food groups high in salt

Food	Salt content
Bread	Each serving may not contain a lot of salt, but it is easy to eat several portions of bread a day
Cold cuts	One 50 g serving, or 6 thin slices, of cured deli meats can contain as much as half your daily recommended dietary salt.
Pizza	A slice of pizza with several toppings can contain more than half your daily recommended dietary salt.
Poultry	Poultry can contain a lot of salt. It depends on how the food was prepared. Read the labels on the packaging carefully.
Soup	Canned soup can contain more than half your daily recommended dietary salt. Check the label carefully before eating.
Sandwiches	A shop-bought sandwich or fast food burger can contain more than your daily recommended dietary salt. Try eating half a sandwich with a side salad instead.

Source Adapted from AHA recommendations.

Salt is used by the food manufacturing industry as both a preservative and cheap ingredient for adding taste. To lower salt intake at the population level, government policies must encourage the food and restaurant industry to reduce salt in the food manufacturing process and improve food labelling. At an individual level, a low-salt diet can be achieved by reducing dependency on processed foods, preparing fresh meals at home and shifting to a diet consisting of natural foods such as spinach, beans and pulses that are low in sodium and high in potassium.

Other tips to reduce salt

People often use salt out of habit, but, as well as not adding salt to your meals, you can consider the following tips.

- If you love a salty flavour to your foods, try using a small sprinkling of a low-sodium salt substitute. The long-term aim, though, should be to focus on enjoying other flavours so that you no longer crave salt.
- Reduce your consumption of processed and pre-packaged foods.
- When you must buy processed and pre-packaged foods, look for 'low-salt' or 'sodium-free' on the label. 'Low-salt' foods contain

0.25 grams of salt per 100 grams of food; 'medium-salt' foods contain 0.25–1.25 grams per 100 grams; and 'high-salt' foods contain 1.25 grams or more of salt.

- If the label doesn't state the amount of salt in a particular food, look at the list of ingredients. The closer salt is to the top of the list, the more salt is contained in the food.
- Use only a very small amount of sea salt or rock salt in baking and cooking – or better still, eliminate it altogether.
- Herbs and spices can provide extra flavour, as can seasonings. Examples are ginger, lime juice, lemon juice, garlic and chilli.
- Ketchup, pickled items, mustard, yeast extract and stock cubes can contain high levels of salt. Look for low-salt alternatives.
- Avoid smoked meat and fish, which are high in salt.
- Use a 'low-salt' cookbook or surf the internet for low-salt recipes.
- If the food label gives the sodium content instead of the salt content, multiply the figure by 2.5 to find out the salt content.

Don't be too hyper-vigilant about the exact amount of salt you eat. Just aiming to eat whole, fresh and pre-packaged foods with the lowest salt content and sticking closely to the advice above should make a great difference. You may find your food tastes bland at first, but adding herbs and spices will make meals more interesting and you will find that your taste buds quickly adjust.

Potassium-rich diet

A low potassium intake is associated with an increased risk of high blood pressure and stroke. Although we don't fully understand the mechanism by which potassium lowers blood pressure – it is thought to involve reduced sodium uptake by the kidneys – a diet rich in potassium does protect against the development of high blood pressure, so increasing our intake of potassium-rich foods is a good idea. The typical western diet is high in sodium and low in potassium; both these factors promote the development of high blood pressure. The best way to increase potassium intake is to eat more fresh fruit and vegetables. Foods rich in potassium include apples, apricots, bananas, broccoli, carrots, oranges, potatoes, prunes, spinach, and watermelon.

Alcohol and hypertension

Alcohol has been a socially acceptable relaxant ever since humans first brewed grapes, promoting warmth and enjoyment. Sadly, though, alcohol abuse is a huge problem in Europe and the USA, with one in four adults frequently drinking quantities of alcohol that can be dangerous to their health. A high level of alcohol intake significantly increases blood pressure. People who drink more than two alcoholic drinks a day have double the incidence of hypertension compared to non-drinkers. However, reducing alcohol intake in people with hypertension has been shown to lower blood pressure on average by 4/2 mmHg. Therefore, it is recommended that men with hypertension have no more than two alcoholic drinks a day, while women should not drink more than one alcoholic drink a day. The NHS recommends a maximum of three to four units of alcohol a day in men and two to three units a day in women (Table 13).

- 1 unit of alcohol is equivalent to 10 ml, or 8 grams, of pure alcohol.
- 1 standard glass of wine = 2 units
- 1 shot of spirits = 1 unit
- 1 pint or can of standard lager or beer = 2 units.

Table 13 Summary of lifestyle changes that should reduce your blood pressure

Lifestyle change	Target	Typical systolic blood pressure reduction (mmHg)
Weight loss	BMI 18.5–25 kg/m² or 5–10 kg weight loss	20
Exercise	30 minutes of aerobic exercise five times per week	4–9
Dietary sodium	Aim for 2.3 grams of sodium or 6 grams salt per day reduction	2–8
Reduce alcohol intake	Up to 2 drinks for men or 1 for women per day (21 units men/14 units women per week)	2–4

Smoking

Cigarette smoking causes a small, chronic elevation in blood pressure seen on ABPM, and an acute rise in blood pressure after a cigarette due to the stimulating effects of nicotine. The major harm from smoking comes from hardening of the arteries and the increased risk of heart attack. People with hypertension are already at increased risk of heart disease and stroke, and smoking escalates the risk several fold. The toxic substances in cigarette smoke cause an accelerated build-up of fatty plaques in the walls of arteries that are already under increased strain due to high blood pressure. Smoking also makes the blood more likely to clot, which is one reason why people have a heart attack. Stopping smoking will significantly reduce the risk of heart disease and will immediately reverse the increased clotting tendency of the blood. Smoking is also a risk factor for cancer and lung damage leading to emphysema – along with other health dangers, of course.

Some facts about smoking addiction

- In the UK smoking is the main cause of preventable disease and death.
- 87 per cent of lung cancers are due to smoking.
- Most cases of emphysema and chronic bronchitis are due to smoking.
- There are 43 distinct cancer-causing chemicals in cigarettes.
- In the UK 30–40 per cent of all deaths from heart disease are directly related to smoking.
- The younger you are when you start smoking, the more likely you are to die prematurely from a smoking-related disease.
- People who smoke 20 cigarettes a day die, on average, seven years earlier than people who have never smoked.
- People who smoke 20 cigarettes a day have more than double the risk of heart attack than non-smokers.
- Smokers who have a heart attack are more likely to die within an hour of the attack than non-smokers.
- A person who successfully stops smoking has the same risk of heart disease 15 years later as a lifelong non-smoker.

How smoking affects the body

The main diseases related to smoking are heart disease, stroke, vascular disease, cancer and lung problems, such as emphysema (the abnormal dilation of air spaces in the lungs) and bronchitis. Smoking can also accelerate osteoporosis, delay the healing of peptic ulcers and cause chronic pains in the legs (claudication), which in severe cases can progress to gangrene and amputation.

- Female smokers are likely to experience an early menopause, while middle-aged and elderly male smokers are likely to suffer from erectile dysfunction.
- Smoking can also lower male fertility and impair female fertility.
- Smokers are two to six times more likely than non-smokers to have coughs, increased phlegm, wheezing and shortness of breath.
- Smoking affects physical appearance, causing bad breath, stained teeth and, sometimes, yellowed finger tips. The skin of a smoker becomes thin and more prone to wrinkling, while the average smoker looks five years older than a non-smoker.
- Smoking during pregnancy adversely affects the developing baby, increasing the risk of abnormal brain development and Sudden Infant Death Syndrome (SIDS).
- Children of parents who both smoke in the house obtain as much nicotine as they would if they smoked 80 cigarettes a year. Hyperactivity and behavioural problems can occur in toddlers.
- The children of smokers are more likely to suffer from chronic respiratory illnesses such as bronchitis, pneumonia and asthma.

Smoking and high blood pressure

Smokers with high blood pressure are likely to see their blood pressure rising further and eventually progress to heart disease. The risk of developing heart disease increases alarmingly in relation to the amount someone smokes, so that, for example, someone who smokes 40 cigarettes a day stands a far greater chance of heart attack than someone who smokes 10 a day. Nicotine is a vasoconstrictor, which means that it narrows arteries and blood vessels, meaning that the heart must work harder to pump blood through them, causing the heart muscle to become enlarged. Smoking affects arteries and blood vessels in the following ways.

- The carbon monoxide from smoking decreases levels of good cholesterol (HDL) in the blood and raises levels of bad cholesterol (LDL), causing cholesterol deposits to form on blood vessel walls. This gradually constricts the arteries and other blood vessels, and once again the heart must work harder and faster to push blood through.
- A lack of oxygen in the body works with nicotine to make the blood vessels too thin. When a blood vessel in the heart bursts, the immediate outcome is a heart attack. When a blood vessel in the head bursts, the immediate outcome is a stroke.
- High levels of nicotine in the body can cause blood clots to form. If immediate help is not sought, this often results in a heart attack or stroke.

Stopping smoking

Side effects of smoking cessation include restlessness, irritability, poor concentration, mood swings, increased appetite, light-headedness, nocturnal waking and cravings. You can expect these side effects to last for two to four weeks, with the exception of an increased appetite which can last two to three months. These are some tips to help you stop smoking.

- Set a date for smoking your last cigarette. Try to choose a day that is generally stress-free but also gives you a chance to keep yourself busy.
- Ask your doctor for help and advice. Nicotine replacement therapy may be useful, as may your local NHS anti-smoking clinic. Get a free *Quit Smoking* support pack and DVD from the NHS Smoking Helpline website, which has useful resources and advice.
- Get support from organizations such as QUIT.
- Relapses are most likely in the first week after quitting, but you can restart your week any time. Just keep going.
- If possible, find a friend to quit with you.
- Inform family and friends of your intentions and ask for their support.
- Stay away from people who smoke. Most urges to start smoking again occur when a smoker is present.
- Try and get plenty of exercise and rest before you stop smoking

so you are more relaxed. Drink more fluids and ensure your diet is as healthy as possible.

- Avoid smoking triggers as much as possible, such as fellow smokers or places where you used to smoke.
- Try the deep breathing routine (described later on in this chapter) when tempted to light up. Bear in mind that a craving doesn't usually last for more than three to five minutes.

Stress

The stress response is encoded into our physical make-up. Acute stress can have a significant impact upon the body with the release of stress hormones such as adrenaline and cortisol, which prepare the body either to fight or to run away, the 'fight or flight' response. The result is a sudden increase in blood pressure due to constriction of blood vessels and increased heart rate and contraction. This physiological response is useful if we are under physical threat but not helpful in dealing with stressful events of modern life. Fortunately, such changes are short lived and blood pressure quickly returns to baseline levels. It is not clear whether chronic stress can result in persistent elevation in blood pressure and hypertension. What is certain is that having coping strategies to manage stress can improve health and wellbeing.

What is stress?

Stress is the feeling we get when we are unable to cope anymore, due to too much mental or emotional pressure. Common symptoms include anxiety, irritability, frequent headaches, palpitations, a feeling of isolation from family and friends, poor sleep and even depression. Unfortunately, many people who are stressed seek false remedies in the form of alcohol, smoking, over-eating and becoming less active than normal – all behaviours guaranteed to make high blood pressure worse, along with its associated health risks.

Stress management strategies

As well as coping with stress itself, aim to make lifestyle changes that stop your body from reacting to stress in the first place.

- Ensure you get plenty of exercise. Sustained, daily, gentle exercise, for example walking, is an effective stress deterrent. Gentle yoga and gardening are also good.
- Do less. If you feel rushed all the time, cut down on activities or space them out, prioritising those that are important to you.
- Learn to say 'no', especially when you're asked to do something that you know you will find stressful.
- Cultivate supportive friends, and gently distance those who take without giving in return.
- Listen to music. Music is a great tension-reliever and can lower blood pressure, relax the body and calm the mind. Singing is effective, too.
- Laughter is a good way to banish stress. Talk to a friend you know you can share a joke with, or watch a funny film.
- Write a diary. Writing down your thoughts can clarify and minimise problems, and help you think of solutions.
- Try to get enough sleep. Again, exercise is helpful with this.
- Watch your breathing (see the deep breathing exercise described in the next section).
- Research has shown that a cluttered environment can cause extra stress, so keep your living and working space tidy. Have a clear out if you need to.
- Try and accept you are not always in control. While it is a good idea to focus on finding solutions, rather than complaining, it isn't always possible to get life perfect. If you have made all the recommended changes to your lifestyle and your blood pressure remains stubbornly high, don't blame yourself – you have done all you can. It is a fact that some people can only lower their blood pressure by taking medication.

Using deep breathing

When we are stressed or upset we breathe more quickly, using the rib muscles rather than the diaphragm to expand the chest so we also breathe more shallowly. This is fine in an emergency as it results in a rush of extra oxygen, providing our bodies with the extra power needed to handle the crisis. Chest-breathing can become a habit in some people, however, which can impact on their physical and emotional health, often causing hyperventilation, panic attacks, chest pains and dizziness. This is a deep breathing exercise that, ideally, you should perform daily.

1 Make yourself comfortable in a warm room where you know you will be alone for at least half an hour.
2 Close your eyes and try to relax.
3 Gradually slow down your breathing, inhaling and exhaling as evenly as possible.
4 Place one hand on your chest and the other on your abdomen, just below your rib-cage.
5 As you inhale, allow your abdomen to swell upward (your chest should barely move).
6 As you exhale, let your abdomen flatten.
7 Give yourself a few minutes to get into a smooth, easy rhythm. As worries and distractions arise, don't hang on to them. Wait calmly for them to float out of your mind – then focus once more on your breathing.
8 When you feel ready to end the exercise, open your eyes. Allow yourself time to become alert before rolling on to one side and getting up. With practice, you will begin breathing with your diaphragm quite naturally – and in times of stress, you should be able to correct your breathing without too much effort.

Better sleep

Getting a good night's sleep is vital to restore energy and help us to cope with stress. For sounder sleep, try the following tips.

- No caffeine after 4 p.m., or after 2 p.m., if you are very sensitive to its effects – caffeine is a stimulant found in coffee, tea, cola drinks and chocolate.
- Use your bedroom only for sleeping – don't watch TV, use computers or your mobile phone in it.
- Ensure that the bedroom is not too hot.
- Establish a bedtime routine and aim to go to bed at the same time every night.
- A quiet period before bedtime – reading a book or listening to music – helps you to calm down in preparation for sleep. Ideally, though, this quiet period should be part of a relatively calm and unhurried lifestyle. Trying to cram too much into the day, with too much stimulus from people and activities, is not always conducive to sleep.
- Have a warm bath, followed by a warm milky drink, before going to bed.
- If your mind is running away with thoughts, write them down.
- When you just can't get to sleep, don't lie there tossing and turning. Get up, make yourself a warm milky drink and try reading a dull book or tackling a routine chore such as paying bills.
- If you suspect that the medication you are taking interferes with your sleep, tell your doctor. There is likely to be an alternative drug he or she can prescribe.
- If you can't get enough sleep no matter what you try, ask your doctor for advice or referral to a sleep clinic.

10

Five steps to improve blood pressure control

The AHA has advocated five simple steps that anyone with hypertension can follow to improve blood pressure control.

1 Know your target

The target blood pressure for most people with high blood pressure is a systolic pressure below 140 and a diastolic pressure below 90. If you have hypertension, you should aim to achieve satisfactory blood pressure levels with a combination of lifestyle changes and intensification of drug treatment, if required. It is not enough simply to take hypertension drug treatment without having a blood pressure goal.

2 Make a plan

High blood pressure is silent. Over the long term it will increase the risk of serious cardiovascular complications such as stroke, heart attacks and aortic aneurysms. Therefore, it is important to diagnose hypertension by having your blood pressure checked even if you feel well. Patients at most risk are those over the age of 40, who are diabetic or known to have kidney disease. Treatment for hypertension is a long-term strategy with the aim of preventing complications. It is important to discuss treatment options with your physician and consider the following questions.

- What stage of hypertension do I have?
- What is my 10-year risk of cardiovascular complications taking into account all cardiovascular risk factors including cholesterol, smoking and family history?
- Are there any potential secondary causes for hypertension?
- Do I need to take medications and if so which ones?

- What are the potential complications of treatment?
- How will I know if the medications are working or if I need to change them?

3 Make a few lifestyle changes

Obesity is a major risk factor for hypertension and our target BMI is 19–25 kg/m^2. In overweight patients, a 10 kg weight loss will result in a reduction in blood pressure by approximately 10 mmHg. This may be enough to lower blood pressure to a normal range and avoid the need to take blood pressure drugs. A diet rich in vegetables, fruit, low-fat diary products and lean protein, such at the DASH diet, can reduce blood pressure by 6–10 mmHg. This diet should be combined with a low salt intake of ideally less than 1.5 grams salt per day, with a reasonable initial target of less than 2.5 grams salt per day. An increase in physical activity with exercise for 30 minutes five times per week will reduce blood pressure and can be achieved using simple changes such as walking to work or taking the stairs instead of the lift. High alcohol intake can exacerbate high blood pressure and you should aim to drink only 1–2 drinks per day (equivalent to 21 units in men and 14 in women per week).

4 Check your blood pressure at home

Automated blood pressure monitors are relatively inexpensive and accurate and can be used to record blood pressure at home. It is important to keep a record of home blood pressure readings, which can be reviewed with your GP to monitor treatment. Home blood pressure readings are more accurate than readings taken at a clinic, will identify those with white coat hypertension, and will allow appropriate adjustment in medication depending on readings. Actively monitoring your blood pressure also encourages better compliance with drug treatment and adds motivation to engage in appropriate lifestyle changes.

5 Take your medication as prescribed

You should be clear what dose and frequency of medications you have been prescribed to treat high blood pressure. Any possible side effects that may interfere with treatment need to be discussed with your GP, who will consider alternatives. Discontinuation of drug therapy can result in uncontrolled high blood pressure levels that may have serious complications and should only be undertaken after talking to your GP. Inadequate blood pressure control increases long-term risk, and the leading cause for failure to achieve blood pressure targets is non-compliance with drug treatment.

Conclusion

This is a brief summary of the important points discussed in the book.

- Hypertension is a very common condition that affects one in three adults in Europe and the USA.
- It is the number one global cause of premature death and the number of people with high blood pressure is likely to increase by 50 per cent over the next two decades.
- Untreated high blood pressure is a major risk factor for stroke, kidney failure, coronary artery disease and heart failure.
- High blood pressure is silent and the only way to diagnose hypertension is to have your blood pressure measured. It is estimated that one-third of all people with high blood pressure are undiagnosed due to inadequate blood pressure screening in the general population.
- You are more at risk if you are over 40, overweight, have a family history of high blood pressure, have chronic kidney disease and/ or a history of cardiovascular disease.
- Most cases of hypertension are due to a combination of genetic and lifestyle factors with no single underlying cause (primary hypertension). Around 10 per cent of all cases have a specific cause for high blood pressure (secondary hypertension), which if treated can reduce blood pressure back down to near normal levels.
- There is general agreement among the international medical community that a systolic blood pressure more than 140 mmHg or diastolic more than 90 mmHg is considered as hypertension.
- Target treatment level is a systolic pressure of less than 140 mmHg (or less than 150 mmHg for people aged over 80) and diastolic less than 90 mmHg.
- Treatment consists of targeting all cardiovascular risk factors, lifestyles changes and appropriate drug therapy.
- Lifestyle changes combined can have a significant impact in lowering blood pressure (exercise, the DASH diet, low sodium-high potassium diet and weight reduction).

- The benefits of drug therapy are due to blood pressure reduction and not due to any intrinsic superiority of one drug over another. Blood-pressure lowering drug therapy had been shown to significantly reduce cardiovascular risk and prolong survival (the drugs do work!).
- 24-hour AMBP monitoring and HBPM are increasingly useful tools to confirm diagnosis of true hypertension and monitor treatment.
- The BHS/NICE four-step algorithm for drug initiation and titration is simple and easy to follow to decide on which class of hypertension drugs to use.
- Blood pressure control is poor with around half of all patients failing to achieve a target blood pressure of less than 140/90.
- Multiple factors are likely to be contributing to poor blood pressure treatment including inadequate patient education, poor compliance with medication, unhealthy lifestyle choices and failure to increase drug therapy in resistant cases.
- Of patients started on drug treatment for hypertension, 35 per cent will stop treatment within 2 years.
- To improve compliance it is important to support and provide education for patients with increased use of HBPM.
- Secondary forms of hypertension need to be considered in cases of resistant or difficult to control hypertension.
- Patients with hard to treat hypertension should be considered for referral to specialist hypertension clinics. Most patients can be managed in primary care.

Case studies

John, a 62-year-old sales manager
John sees his GP for a routine check-up and is found to have a blood pressure of 164/104 mmHg. His GP repeats this after John has rested and records a similar second reading. John has no previous medical problems. He doesn't smoke, is slightly overweight and is not on any regular medication. He drinks approximately 14 units of alcohol per week (which is within the recommended range for men). There is a history of heart disease in his family, as his father had a heart attack in his 50s.

What does John's GP do next?
John's GP recommends that he has ambulatory blood pressure monitoring to exclude white coat hypertension and to enable a more accurate assessment of blood pressure levels. He goes on to have this and it shows that John's daytime average blood pressure is 148/104 mmHg. John's GP is also interested in the possibility that there could be an underlying medical reason for John's high blood pressure. Therefore, John also has blood tests and a urine check. John's GP examines the back of his eyes (his retinas), which show no signs of damage from high blood pressure. An ECG is performed: this is also normal and does not show abnormally increased thickness of the heart muscle.

What do the test results show?
The tests confirm that John has stage 2 hypertension. John wants to know why he has high blood pressure; his GP explains that 90 per cent of all hypertension has no single identifiable cause and often occurs because of lifestyle and genetic factors. John's GP prescribes John a drug for his hypertension and gives him some lifestyle advice. John is advised to lose some weight, as on average, a 10 kg weight loss results in 10 mmHg reduction in systolic blood pressure. John is encouraged to eat a low-salt diet (less than 6 grams salt or 2.5 grams of sodium a day) and do 30 minutes of aerobic exercise five times a week. For the drug treatment, John's GP prescribes a calcium-channel blocker, amlodipine, at a dosage of 5 mg. After 2 weeks on the drug, John goes back to see his doctor. His blood pressure is now 154/96 mmHg.

Is the treatment working?
John's GP is aiming for a blood pressure of less than 140/90 mmHg. John's blood pressure is currently higher than that so his GP has to

decide whether to increase the dose of amlodipine, switch to a different drug, or prescribe a second drug to be taken with the amlodipine. John's GP decides to increase the dose of amlodipine from 5 mg to 10 mg daily. Unfortunately, John develops swollen ankles and headaches on the higher dose and stops taking the drugs. Instead of increasing the dose of amlodipine to 10 mg (which can be associated with more side effects such as ankle swelling), another option would have been to add in a second drug to amlodipine to improve John's blood pressure.

Trevor, a 54-year-old professional sports commentator

Trevor has been on treatment for high blood pressure for the last 4 years after a minor stroke that affected his speech. He does not smoke and rarely drinks alcohol. His GP gives him a check-up, which is normal apart from his blood pressure which is 154/96.

Trevor is currently taking three blood pressure drugs at reasonable doses: a calcium-channel blocker, thiazide diuretic and an ACE inhibitor. He is referred to the blood pressure clinic at his local hospital for further investigation.

What is Trevor's diagnosis?

The doctor at the clinic suggests that Trevor has resistant hypertension, as the drug treatment is not lowering Trevor's blood pressure. The doctors suggests that Trevor does 24-hour ambulatory blood pressure monitoring to rule out white coat hypertension; this shows a mean daytime blood pressure of 150/93 mmHg. Blood tests show that Trevor's kidneys are working properly; the urine dipstick test is normal with no detectable blood or protein. However, an ECG shows evidence of left ventricular hypertrophy (or thickness in his heart muscle).

What treatment is available?

Trevor has true resistant hypertension, confirmed by ambulatory blood pressure monitoring, evidence of target organ damage from his previous stroke and the ECG showing left ventricular hypertrophy. The doctor at the clinic arranges an echocardiogram to define the extent of heart wall thickness. This confirms that all of Trevor's left ventricle has become moderately thick. Spironolactone is recommended for resistant hypertension in patients like Trevor. However, despite Trevor taking spironolactone alongside his other blood pressure drugs, his blood pressure remains above 140/90.

Is the treatment working?

When Trevor returns to the clinic, he reports symptoms that could mean that he has obstructive sleep apnoea: snoring, daytime sleepiness, morning headaches, memory impairment and poor concentration.

His wife says that he often appears to choke or gasp during his sleep. Trevor's doctor refers him for sleep studies, in which his oxygen levels are measured as he sleeps, along with his heart rate and breathing. These tests confirm that Trevor has episodes of interrupted breathing during sleep and he is diagnosed with obstructive sleep apnoea. The treatment for obstructive sleep apnoea includes avoiding both alcohol and night-time sedatives. Trevor is taught how to use a CPAP machine, which has a tight fitting nasal mask with a continuous airflow that prevents obstruction of his airway while he sleeps. This treatment results in Trevor's blood pressure being lowered to target levels, and illustrates that obstructive sleep apnoea is one of the most common causes of resistant hypertension.

Useful addresses

UK-based organizations

Blood Pressure Association
60 Cranmer Terrace
London SW17 0QS
Tel.: 020 8772 4994
Blood Pressure Information Line: 0845 241 0989 (11 a.m. to 3 p.m., Monday to Friday)
Website: www.bpassoc.org.uk
The only UK-wide charity that focuses solely on tackling high blood pressure. Offers a range of information and support to help people take control of, or avoid, this condition.

British Heart Foundation
Greater London House
180 Hampstead Road
London NW1 7AW
Tel.: 020 7554 0000 (9 a.m. to 5 p.m., Monday to Friday)
Heart HelpLine: 0300 330 3311 (9 a.m. to 6 p.m., Monday to Friday)
Website: www.bhf.org.uk
Provides a range of information about the causes, prevention and treatment of heart disease. There is also a glossary and details of publications, plus practical advice on how to protect yourself from heart disease.

British Hypertension Society
Website: www.bhsoc.org
For professional enquiries about information on hypertension write to:
Jackie Howarth
BHS Administrative Officer
Clinical Sciences Building
Level 5
Leicester Royal Infirmary
PO Box 65
Leicester LE2 7LX
Tel.: 07717 467 973

For enquiries about meetings, membership etc. write to:
Mrs Gerry McCarthy
Meetings Secretary
Hampton Medical Conferences Ltd
113–119 High Street
Hampton Hill
Middlesex TW12 1NJ
Tel.: 020 8979 8300
Website: www.hamptonmedical.com
Provides a medical and scientific research forum to enable sharing of cutting-edge research, to understand the origin of high blood pressure and improve its treatment.

High Blood Pressure Foundation
Department of Medical Sciences
Western General Hospital
Edinburgh EH4 2XU
Tel.: 0131 332 9211
Website: www.hbpf.org.uk
Aims to improve the basic understanding, assessment, treatment and public awareness of high blood pressure, and in so doing help promote the welfare of people with the condition.

NHS Direct
Helpline: 0845 4647 (24 hours a day)
Website: www.nhsdirect.nhs.uk
This 24-hour NHS service provides expert health advice from trained nurses. An extensive database of medical information is available on the website. The nurses can also advise you if you wish to make a complaint about the NHS.

NHS Smoking Helpline
Tel.: 0800 022 4332 (7 a.m. to 11 p.m., 7 days a week)
Website: www.nhs.uk/smokefree
A website giving support and advice on how to quit smoking, with information on local-group sessions, a programme giving support at home and advice on how nicotine replacement products can help you to manage cravings.

QUIT
63 St Mary's Axe
London EC3A 8AA
Tel.: 020 7469 0400
Quitline: 0800 00 22 00 (for free, individual, same-day advice from
trained counsellors)
Website: www.quit.org.uk
The aim of QUIT is to significantly reduce unnecessary suffering and
death from smoking-related diseases. It provides practical help, advice and
support to smokers who wish to stop.

Sleep Matters
Tel.: 020 8994 9874 (6 p.m. to 8 p.m., 7 days a week)
Website: www.medicaladvisoryservice.org.uk/html/sleep_matters.html
A nurse-run information line operated by the Medical Advisory Service.
For help and advice on overcoming insomnia and achieving a good
night's sleep.

Stress Management Society
Tel.: 0844 357 8629
Website: www.stress.org.uk

The Stroke Association
Stroke House
240 City Road
London EC1V 2PR
Tel.: 020 7566 0300
Stroke Helpline: 0845 3033 100 (9 a.m. to 5 p.m., Monday to Friday)
Website: www.stroke.org.uk
A non-profit organization dedicated to helping people tackle stress.
Provides information and support for people affected by stroke.

Outside the UK

American Heart Association
National Center
7272 Greenville Avenue
Dallas, TX 75231
Tel.: 1 800 242 8721
Website: www.americanheart.org
For a wealth of information, tools and resources about cardiovascular
disease and stroke, to help you manage your health.

Blood Pressure Canada
Website: www.hypertension.ca
A web-based non-profit charitable organization dedicated to the prevention and control of hypertension (high blood pressure). The organization strives to increase awareness about the condition and reduce the burden of cardiovascular disease.

References

1   Go AS, Mozaffarian D, Roger VL et al. Heart disease and stroke sta-
    tistics – 2013 update: a report from the American Heart Association.
    Circulation 2013; **127**:e6–245.
2   Dahlöf B, Sever PS, Poulter NR et al. Prevention of cardiovascular events
    with an antihypertensive regimen of amlodipine adding perindopril as
    required vs. atenolol adding bendroflumethiazide as required, in the
    Anglo-Scandinavian Cardiac Outcomes Trial-Blood Pressure Lowering
    Arm (ASCOT-BPLA): a multicentre randomised controlled trial. *Lancet*
    2005; **366**: 895–906.
3   Williams B, Lacy PS, Thom SM et al. Differential impact of blood pres-
    sure-lowering drugs on central aortic pressure and clinical outcomes:
    principal results of the Conduit Artery Function Evaluation (CAFE)
    study. *Circulation* 2006; **113**: 1213–25.
4   James PA, Oparil S, Carter BL et al. 2014 Evidence-Based Guideline for
    the Management of High Blood Pressure in Adults: report from the
    panel members appointed to the eighth joint national committee (JNC
    8). *Journal of the American Medical Association* 2014; **311**: 507–20.
5   Chobanian AV, Bakris GL, Black HR et al. The seventh report of the
    Joint National Committee on prevention, detection, evaluation, and
    treatment of high blood pressure: the JNC 7 report. *Journal of the
    American Medical Association* 2003; **289**(19): 2560–72.
6   Mancia G, Fagard R, Narkiewicz K et al. ESH/ESC guidelines for the
    management of arterial hypertension: the Task Force for the manage-
    ment of arterial hypertension of the European Society of Hypertension
    (ESH) and of the European Society of Cardiology (ESC). *European Heart
    Journal* 2013; **34**(28): 2159–219.
7   Stone NJ, Robinson J, Lichtenstein AH et al. 2013 ACC/AHA guide-
    line on the treatment of blood cholesterol to reduce atherosclerotic
    cardiovascular risk in adults: a report of the American College of
    Cardiology/American Heart Association task force on practice guide-
    lines. *Circulation* 2013. Available at: <http://circ.ahajournals.org/
    content/early/2013/11/11/01.cir.0000437738.63853.7a.citation>.
8   Law MR, Morris JK and Wald NJ. Use of blood pressure lowering drugs
    in the prevention of cardiovascular disease: meta-analysis of 147
    randomised trials in the context of expectations from prospective epi-
    demiological studies. *British Medical Journal* 2009; **338**: b1665.
9   Freis ED. The Veterans Administration Cooperative Study on antihy-
    pertensive agents. Implications for stroke prevention. *Stroke* 1974; **5**:
    76–7.
10 Makani H, Bangalore S, Supariwala A et al. Antihypertensive efficacy of
    angiotensin receptor blockers as monotherapy as evaluated by ambula-

tory blood pressure monitoring: a meta-analysis. *European Heart Journal* 2014; **35**: 1732–42.

11 Musini VM, Nazer M, Bassett K et al. Blood pressure-lowering efficacy of monotherapy with thiazide diuretics for primary hypertension. *Cochrane Database of Systematic Reviews* 2014: Issue **5**.

12 Izzo JL, Weintraub HS, Duprez DA et al. Treating systolic hypertension in the very elderly with valsartan-hydrochlorothiazide vs either mono-therapy: ValVET primary results. *The Journal of Clinical Hypertension* 2011; **13**(10): 722–30.

13 National Institute for Health and Care Excellence. Hypertension: Clinical management of primary hypertension in adults (CG127). Available at: <www.nice.org. uk/guidance/cg127>.

14 Dahlöf B, Devereux RB, Kjeldsen SE et al. LIFE Study Group. Cardiovascular morbidity and mortality in the Losartan Intervention For Endpoint reduction in hypertension study (LIFE): a randomised trial against atenolol. *Lancet* 2002; **359**: 995–1003.

15 Go AS, Bauman MA, King SMC et al. An effective approach to high blood pressure control. *Journal of the American College of Cardiology* 2014; **63**: 1230–8.

16 Bhatt DL, Kandzari DE, O'Neill WW et al. A controlled trial of renal denervation for resistant hypertension. *The New England Journal of Medicine* 2014; **370**: 1393–401.

Index